FROM THE EDITORS OF

ESSENCE®

The Black Woman's Guide to
Healthy Living

THE BEST ADVICE FOR BODY, MIND + SPIRIT
IN YOUR 20s, 30s, 40s, 50s + BEYOND

ESSENCE

Editor-in-Chief: Angela Burt-Murray
Executive Editor: Dawn M. Baskerville
Creative Director: Lisa Hunt
Deputy Editor: Rosemarie Robotham
Senior Editor, Health and Relationships: Lynya Floyd
Senior Writer: Jeannine Amber
Associate Art Director: Pinda Diarrassouba-Romain
Research Chief: Christine Gordon
Design Production Manager: LaToya N. Valmont
Associate Photo Editor: Tracey Woods

Book Credits

Text: Robin D. Stone
Design: Alisha Neumaier
Research: Eboni Barnes, Qimmah Saafir
Copyediting: Kenyatta Matthews, Hope Wright
Production: Carina A. Rosario

Content Credits

ESSENCE would like to acknowledge
and thank all the writers who contributed to
and inspired content within this book:
Jennifer Abbasi, Nicole Alper, Jeannine Amber,
Sharon Boone, Joy Buchanan, Michelle Burford,
Margarette Burnette, Claudia Caruana, Julia Chance,
Andrea King Collier, Jessica Cumberbatch, Lynya Floyd,
Nikitta A. Foston, Stacy Gilliam, Lambeth Hochwald,
Tracy E. Hopkins, LaShieka Purvis Hunter,
Hilda Hutcherson, M.D., Tamara Jeffries, Melissa Ewey Johnson,
Tonya Adams Joyner, Ziba Kashef, Nina Malkin,
Claire R. McIntosh, Michele Meyer, Jonell Nash, Leslie O'Hanlon,
Lonnae O'Neal Parker, Leslie Pepper, Rosemarie Robotham,
Nicole Saunders, Markette Smith, Bonnie St. John,
Robin D. Stone, Claire Sulmers, Terrie Williams, Hope Wright

Time Inc. Home Entertainment

Publisher: Richard Fraiman
General Manager: Steven Sandonato
Executive Director, Marketing Services: Carol Pittard
Director, Retail & Special Sales: Tom Mifsud
Director, New Product Development: Peter Harper
Assistant Director, Newsstand Marketing: Laura Adam
Assistant Director, Brand Marketing: Joy Butts
Associate Counsel: Helen Wan
Senior Brand Manager: TWRS/M: Holly Oakes
Brand & Licensing Manager: Alexandra Bliss
Design & Prepress Manager: Ann-Michelle Gallero
Book Production Manager: Susan Chodakiewicz

Special Thanks

Glenn Bunoncore, Margaret Hess, Suzanne Janso,
Brynn Joyce, Robert Marasco,
Brooke Reger, Mary Sarro-Waite, Ilene Schreider,
Adriana Tierno, Alex Voznesenskiy

Copyright 2008
Essence Communications, Inc.
Published by Time Inc. Home
Entertainment

Time Inc.
1271 Avenue of the Americas
New York NY 10020

ISBN 10: 1-60320-043-6
ISBN: 13-978-1-60320-043-1

Printed in Colombia

ESSENCE and ESSENCE Books
are trademarks of
Essence Communications, Inc.

We welcome your comments
and suggestions about ESSENCE Books.
Please write us at:
ESSENCE Books
Attention: Book Editors
P.O. Box 11016
Des Moines IA 50336-1016

If you would like to order any of
our hardcover Collector's Edition books,
please call us at 800-327-6388
(Monday through Friday, 7:00 A.M.–8:00
P.M. or Saturday, 7:00 A.M.–6:00 P.M.,
Central Standard Time)

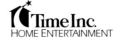

Table of Contents

Keys to Healthy Living }

Like most Americans, Black women work hard.

In fact, we work so hard at our jobs, looking after our families and giving back to our communities that we often ignore our own bodies. We would never neglect to schedule an annual check up for our children, encourage an elder to see a specialist or accompany a loved one to a medical appointment. Yet we often cancel, or worse, never even schedule, routine care for ourselves. We're always putting ourselves last. But the truth is, we're cheating ourselves and shortchanging those who love us. That's why we created this book just for you. *The Black Woman's Guide to Healthy Living* offers comprehensive advice on taking care of your mind, body and spirit. With expert insights, wisdom from women who've been where you are, medical checklists, fun fitness workouts, mental health recommendations and quick and healthy recipes, this book is chock-full of the information you need to gain control of your life. Just follow our lead, and we promise you'll soon be feeling as great as you look. And you'll live longer.

Here are three of my personal tips to get you started on your journey to good health and happiness:

1. **Call the doctor.** Take a personal day to attend to all your annual medical appointments. Follow up on any instructions you may receive from your doctor, and be sure to schedule checkups for the same time next year.

2. **Eat better.** Save time by ordering groceries online; buy organic when possible and eat three balanced meals a day. Treat yourself to colorful snacks—fruits and veggies are rich in nutrients and boost energy and balance mood.

3. **Get moving.** Incorporate exercise into your routine at least three times a week. Even if it's just climbing the stairs instead of riding the elevator or walking around your office building during lunch, every step counts.

We hope this book will inspire you to pay more attention to your own needs as you begin caring for the most important person in your life—you!

Angela

Angela Burt-Murray
Editor-in-Chief

Mission: Control

Taking charge of your health doesn't have to be in the future. We designed this book to guide you toward the best shape of your life now, in just three steps.

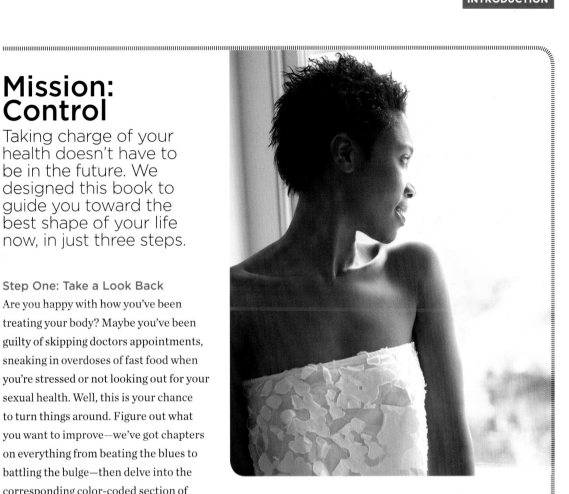

Step One: Take a Look Back

Are you happy with how you've been treating your body? Maybe you've been guilty of skipping doctors appointments, sneaking in overdoses of fast food when you're stressed or not looking out for your sexual health. Well, this is your chance to turn things around. Figure out what you want to improve—we've got chapters on everything from beating the blues to battling the bulge—then delve into the corresponding color-coded section of this book to discover how you can flip your health script.

Step Two: See Where You Stand

Turn to page 8, where we define our health profiles and challenges by the decades. When are you at risk for fibroids? Who should be paying careful attention to that leg cramp? When are you most likely to contract a sexually transmitted infection? Our age-by-age guidelines in this and other sections tell you what to look out for and ask your doctor about.

Step Three: Set Your Sights

What does a healthier you look like in one month? One year? Grab your pen and get ready to shape a whole new you with our personalized food and fitness plan and motivational journal pages. Whether it's figuring out the best way for your friends to support your weight loss endeavors or finally keeping notes on your sleep routines to put an end to tired mornings, everything you need is in your hands.

— **Lynya Floyd, Senior Editor,
Health and Relationships**

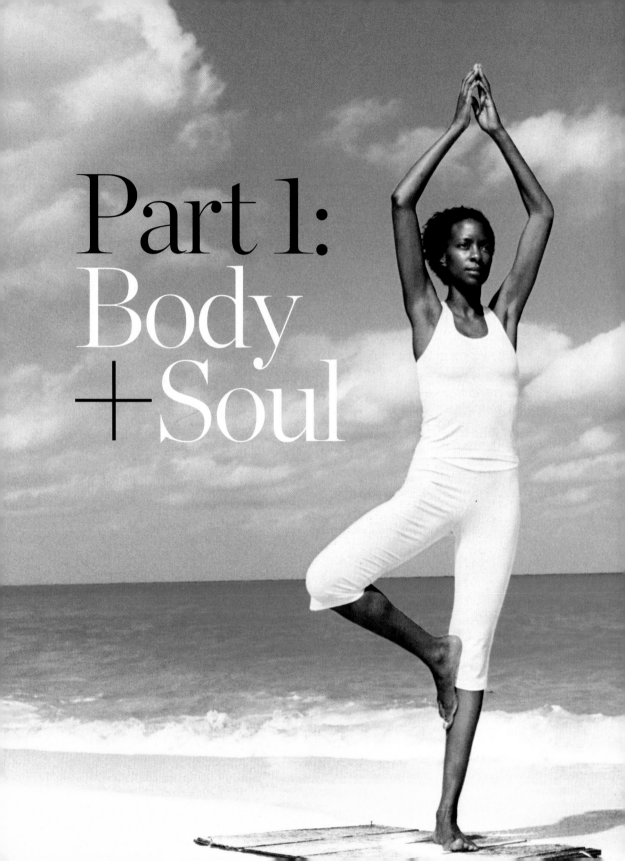

Part 1:
Body
+Soul

Love Your Life

"How are you?"

Three simple words. You probably say them dozens of times each day to other people. But how often do you ask them of yourself? If you're like most Black women, the answer is not enough. You're far too busy taking care of everyone else to focus on your health. But for us, getting healthy needs to be priority number one: African-American women top the charts for life-threatening illnesses like heart disease and cancer. Despite the sobering statistics, once we're informed and motivated, Black women can move mountains. This section will help you do just that. First, take a look at where you stand with our decade-by-decade breakdown of Black women's health. Then delve into our advice from top African-American doctors tackling the critical diseases that affect us. Finally, you'll be able to develop a personalized health action plan with our wellness worksheet. And, every so often, as you make your way through these pages, don't forget to pause and ask yourself, "How am I feeling?" Empowered, we hope. »

Healthy Living at Every Age

You deserve to feel as good as you look. We bring you the experts' take on how to live better in your 20s, 30s, 40s, 50s and beyond. »

20s

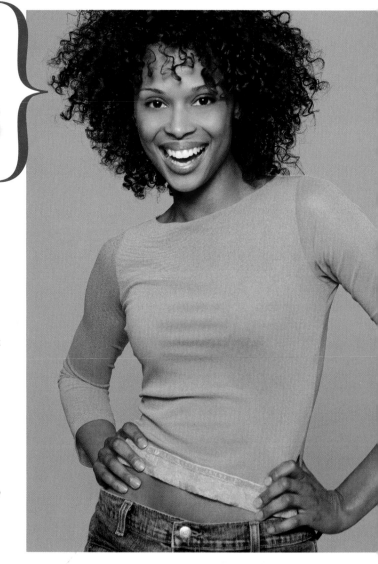

Your Body

Like most women this age, you have stamina to burn and your body is fairly resilient. But if you take that for granted—eating poorly, keeping late hours, not exercising—it will catch up with you. We may be predisposed to illnesses like diabetes or hypertension, but that doesn't mean they are your health destiny. Lay the groundwork for your future by starting healthy habits now.

Your Diet

All that junk food you survived on when you were younger? Time to let it go. Remember these simple food rules to stay fit through the decades:

Eat balanced meals. Be sure to include three to five servings of fruits and vegetables a day. They help keep you regular and they're full of heart-healthy cancer-fighting antioxidants. Eat moderate amounts of lean meats and poultry, and limit sweets and fried foods, to keep your cholesterol down and stave off extra pounds.

Be calcium conscious. Your skeleton will replace itself four to five times during your lifetime, so make sure you're getting enough calcium—1,000 mg per day. Milk, cheese and yogurt will do the trick. If you're lactose intolerant—up to 80 percent of African-Americans are—choose broccoli, fortified soy milk and canned salmon with edible bones.

Drink eight glasses of water daily. It's critical to keep your body hydrated and functioning. Commit to drinking one glass before each meal.

Take a multivitamin. It will help compensate for those times when your diet isn't the best.

Your Fitness

In your twenties, partying usually trumps Pilates, but regular exercise will help you develop the strength, endurance and flexibility that's harder to achieve as you age. Combine cardio, to strengthen your heart and lungs, with weight-resistance, to support the bone mass you're still developing. Mix it up—quick-paced African dance one day, muscle-strengthening yoga another. An hour a day is best, but even a half hour three to five days a week works wonders.

Your Doctor Visits

"A lot of women in their twenties don't think they need regular checkups, but that's a mistake," says Michelle N. Johnson, M.D., assistant chief of cardiology at Memorial Sloan-Kettering Cancer Center in New York. "This is the time to build relationships with doctors you are comfortable with." See your internist, your gynecologist and your dentist annually.

Your Mind + Mood

Life transitions like moving away from home, making new friends, starting a new job, forging business alliances or trying to meet the demands of marriage and motherhood can seem overwhelming. Look to close friends and family members for support. And if you start to experience signs of mental distress, such as sleeplessness, binge eating, social withdrawal or difficulty concentrating, seek professional help.

Your Sexual Health

You're more likely to contract a sexually transmitted infection (STI) during this decade, so make using condoms a top priority. Fifty percent of sexually active women ages 20 to 24 have HPV, and HIV is the leading cause of death for Black women ages 25 to 34. In your twenties, your fertility is peaking. If you're not ready for motherhood, ask your gynecologist to recommend birth control options that match your body and your lifestyle.

Ask Yourself...

WHAT'S MY FAMILY MEDICAL HISTORY?
"Get an idea of the hereditary diseases that may have occurred in family members so that you and your doctors can watch out for warning signs and make lifestyle adjustments where necessary," says Johnny Benjamin, M.D., a spine surgeon and chief of the department of orthopedic surgery at the Indian River Medical Center in Vero Beach, Florida. Feeling ambitious? Interview your relatives and make a family tree tracing illnesses back for generations, then share it with all the branches.

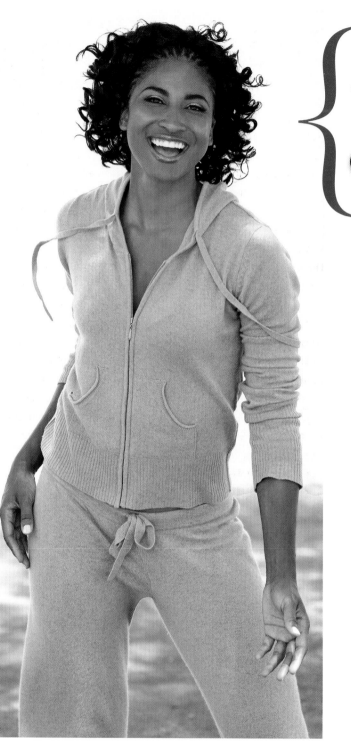

{30s

Your Body

You're super busy making great strides, but you may notice you're gaining weight. "As you age, your metabolism slows down," says Shadrach Smith, M.D., medical director of Hospital Hill Medical Pavilion at Truman Medical Center in Kansas City, Missouri. "This change can result in more total body fat and less muscle mass."

Your Diet

Between work, the kids and family obligations, who's got time to cook a well-balanced meal? "You can always 'assemble' a meal instead," advises Rovenia Brock, Ph.D., author of *Dr. Ro's Ten Secrets to Livin' Healthy* (Bantam). "Throw together a salad. Pop out a prepackaged tuna steak or smoked salmon fillet that's already cooked." If weight is an issue, limit your intake of saturated and processed fats. But don't bypass omega-3s, found in oily varieties of fish, nuts and olive oil. These good fats support cells and cut the risk of cardiovascular ailments. Eat calcium-rich foods for bone health, and dark leafy vegetables to guard against cancer. Consume proper portions, and stop eating three hours before bedtime.

Your Fitness

You're eager to see how far you can still push your body and may be tempted to go to the limit. Or maybe you're too overwhelmed to find time to exercise. Either way, experts recommend balancing cardio and strength training with mind–body exercise. Depending on which form you choose, regular exercise can ease stress-related aches and pains, increase energy and help promote a healthy outlook. Newbies might want to start with a gentle form of yoga. Don't have time for the gym? Pop in an exercise DVD and work out at home, or take a 20-to-30-minute walk before breakfast, during lunch breaks or after dinner.

Your Doctor Visits

You might feel like you have too much going on to see a doctor, but you'll need to make time. Have your thyroid checked to see if it may be overactive (which can make you lose weight, and feel nervous and weak) or underactive (you may feel tired and forgetful, and start gaining weight). "Thyroid disease is one of the most commonly undiagnosed conditions," says Nieca Goldberg, M.D., clinical associate professor and medical director of New York University

Women's Heart Program and author of *Dr. Nieca Goldberg's Complete Guide to Women's Health* (Ballantine Books).

Your Mind + Mood

You can't stop the whirl of your merry-go-round, but you owe it to yourself to step off regularly. Not only are those time-outs emotionally restorative, but they will also keep you sharp when you get back on the ride. "Force yourself each week to engage in one to three activities that you enjoy," says Tené T. Lewis, Ph.D., assistant professor in the department of epidemiology and public health at Yale University School of Medicine. Explore a hobby, read a book, catch up with girlfriends, or just be still and meditate.

Your Sexual Health

If you want a baby, it's time to stop dreaming and start planning. "At age 39, there's a steep drop in women's fertility," points out Hilda Hutcherson, M.D., clinical professor of obstetrics and gynecology at Columbia University Medical Center and the author of *Pleasure: A Woman's Guide to Getting the Sex You Want, Need and Deserve* (Perigee Trade). "You don't have to rush, but you and your partner need to map out a timeline." And be on the lookout for fibroids; they are often found in African-American women in their thirties. "If you're experiencing pain and heavy menstrual bleeding, fibroids could be the likely cause," Hutcherson says.

Ask Yourself...

AM I AT RISK FOR DIABETES?

"Just being African-American is a risk factor for diabetes, but family history, gestational diabetes and excess weight all increase your chances of a diagnosis," says Griffin P. Rodgers, M.D., director of the National Institute of Diabetes and Digestive and Kidney Diseases at the National Institutes of Health. Surprisingly, one third of adults with diabetes don't know they have it. Warning signs include frequent urination, excessive thirst, unusual weight loss, blurred vision and increased fatigue. Ask your doctor about getting a blood glucose test.

40s

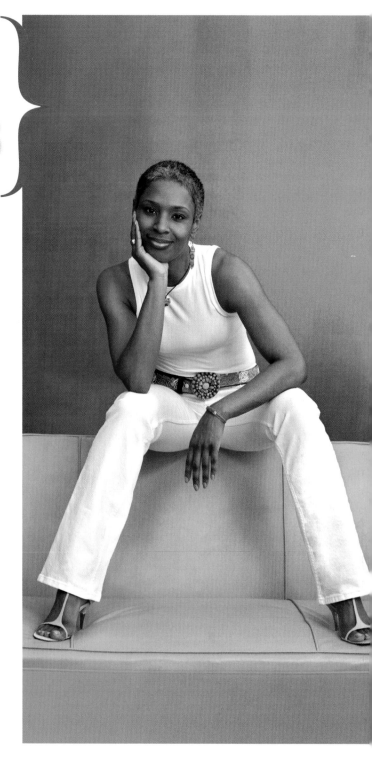

Your Body

You're coming into your own, feeling good about the skin you're in and focused on what you want from life. But there are variables: Feeling moody? Frustrated with irregular periods? Perimenopause, the precursor to menopause, may be kicking in. Weight gain is more prevalent, especially around your middle, predisposing you to diabetes, hypertension and heart disease, which is the number one killer of women. Your vision's also changing, making it more difficult to read small print. "Your body is starting to talk to you now," says Cheryl Rucker-Whitaker, M.D., director of preventive cardiology in the Heart Center for Women at Rush University Hypertension Center in Chicago. Those missed gym dates and indulgent meals may be catching up to you.

Your Diet

If you're still struggling to balance your diet, hone in on natural foods with visual variety. "The more colorful, the better," says Kacy Duke, a celebrity personal trainer, fitness consultant and author of *The Show It Love Workout* (McGraw-Hill). "That lets you know you're getting the right vitamins." Ensure that your meals are full of nutrients by cooking with healthy fats, like olive oil. If your metabolism is slowing down due to menopause, try eating six small meals during the course of the day, recommends Rovenia Brock, Ph.D., author of *Dr. Ro's Ten Secrets to Livin' Healthy* (Bantam). Continue to take in enough calcium, to prevent the onset of osteoporosis, and foods rich in omega-3 fats, to guard against heart disease.

Your Fitness

Whittle that tummy bulge by mixing cardiovascular and toning workouts. "If you have joint problems, avoid high-impact exercises that could cause damage," advises Michele Martin-Jones, M.D., a family physician in Baltimore. Try Pilates, swimming or biking, all of which give you a good workout but are easy on the joints. Strength training is a must now, as a decrease in muscle mass could put you at increased risk of disability. "Women naturally lose about a half pound of muscle every year during their adult life," says Duke. "But you can increase your strength 100 percent in just 12 weeks of strength training."

Your Doctor Visits

These are all the more important because you must catch problems—like breast cancer—as early as possible. Annual mammograms are a priority, says Sydney McCalla, M.D., chief of breast surgery service at Lincoln Hospital in New York.

"When African-American women are diagnosed, they tend to be at a more advanced stage and are more likely to die from the disease," he says. African-American women are particularly vulnerable to rare and aggressive forms of the disease, such as triple negative breast cancer (which isn't fueled by estrogen, progesterone or the HER2 gene) and inflammatory breast cancer (the signs: redness, swelling or tenderness of the breast instead of a lump).

Your Mind + Mood

Your forties can be exciting years as you're more confident and comfortable with yourself and your place in the world. But you're also entering the Sandwich Generation. Perhaps you're juggling motherhood and a career while taking care of elder family members as well as grandchildren. Look to family members or your sister circle of friends for support, or seek professional help.

Your Sexual Health

With the decrease in estrogen that comes during perimenopause, you may experience decreased sex drive along with irregular periods, hot flashes, irritability and problems sleeping. Eat soy-based foods, which may help alleviate symptoms of perimenopause and menopause, and talk to your doctor about treatments that may restore balance. Regular sexual activity now means you'll be less likely to have vaginal dryness in your fifties. Not seeing anyone? Invest in a vibrator or shower massager.

Ask Yourself...

WHY CAN'T I SHAKE THIS BAD MOOD?

"All of us get the blues, but clinical depression stops you in your tracks," says Freida Hopkins Outlaw, assistant commissioner of special populations and minority services at the Tennessee Department of Mental Health and Developmental Disabilities. At midlife, past bouts with depression put us at higher risk of physical and emotional symptoms, which include deep fatigue, social withdrawal, problems concentrating and trouble getting out of bed. "Don't discount what you're feeling," Outlaw says. Admitting that you're depressed is the first step to getting well.

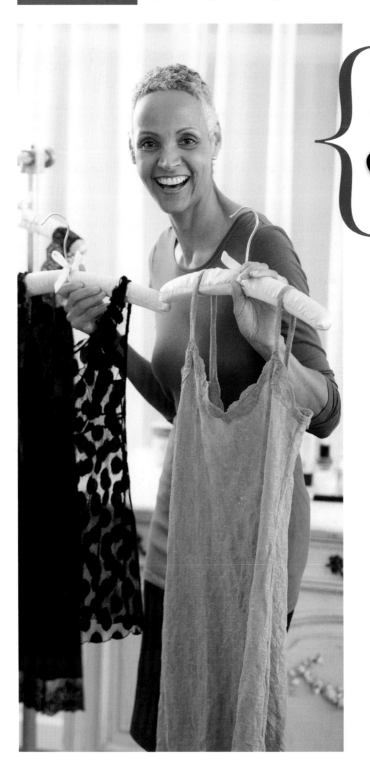

{50s + beyond...

Your Body

They say that 50 is the new 40— that's affirmation of the vitality you can possess at this age and beyond. African-American women are definitely living longer. In 2006, Black women hit a record high life expectancy of 76.9 years. But chronic conditions and physical limitations all increase with age, so it's more important than ever to keep up with preventive doctor visits and follow-up care for any illnesses.

Your Diet

Make sure you're getting enough calcium. "After menopause, the body starts leeching calcium away from the bones," says Johnny Benjamin, M.D., a spine surgeon and chief of the department of orthopedic surgery at the Indian River Medical Center in Vero Beach, Florida. Take a daily calcium supplement with vitamin D, which will help your body absorb the calcium. And fill up on foods rich in fiber: It can help control diabetes and digestive disorders.

Your Fitness

Listen to your body. Since you're more vulnerable to injury as you age, you need to respect your limitations. "Being present in your workout helps you do that," says Kacy Duke, a celebrity personal trainer, fitness consultant and author of *The Show It Love Workout* (McGraw-Hill). She encourages women to turn off the TV when they're working out. Consider gentler forms of exercise, like walking, swimming and tai chi, which can help prevent arthritis, in addition to weight-bearing exercises that can help fight osteoporosis.

Your Doctor Visits

If you're seeing multiple doctors, update them about changes in your health and current medications and treatments (keep a list in your purse). You'll want a bone density test to check for signs of osteoporosis, and schedule a colonoscopy—colon cancer is the third most common form of cancer in African-American women, but thanks to detection tools, rates have dropped. Also be on the lookout for ovarian cancer, which tends to strike after menopause with vague symptoms like abdominal pressure, urinary urgency and pelvic pain.

Your Mind + Mood

Fifties-plus can feel like newfound freedom years. With your children grown and on their own, you can finally shift your focus back to you. Learn a new skill or start a hobby, or sign up for volunteer work. Staying active and engaged can boost both your physical and mental health. Eighteen percent of postmenopausal women experience panic attacks, with symptoms that include a pounding heart, dizziness, shaking and shortness of breath. The symptoms are similar to those of a heart attack and could lead to a misdiagnosis, says Freida Hopkins Outlaw, assistant commissioner of special populations and minority services at the Tennessee Department of Mental Health. If these signs send you to the doctor, perhaps you need a mental health screening in addition to a physical exam.

Your Sexual Health

With no monthly period and no chance of pregnancy, some women feel freer to enjoy sex. But don't forget about safe sex. Fifteen percent of new HIV/AIDS diagnoses are in people ages 50 and up, and rates of HIV/AIDS in Blacks are 12 times as high as among Whites. If menopause results in vaginal dryness and a loss of libido, see a doctor. You can get your groove back. As Hilda Hutcherson, M.D., clinical professor of obstetrics and gynecology at Columbia University Medical Center and the author of *Pleasure: A Woman's Guide to Getting the Sex You Want, Need and Deserve* (Perigee Trade), says, "The good news is women in their fifties are more comfortable telling their partners what they need and want in bed."

Ask Yourself...

AM I HAVING LEG PAINS?

If you experience intense muscle cramps in your calves or muscle pain in your hips or buttocks, you could have peripheral artery disease (PAD), a condition caused by cholesterol buildup in the artery walls. "It's an aggressive condition that can make it hard for you to get around, and it can increase your chances of having a heart attack or stroke," cautions Emile R. Mohler III, M.D., director of vascular medicine for the University of Pennsylvania Health System. African-American women with high blood pressure are especially at risk, so talk to your doctor.

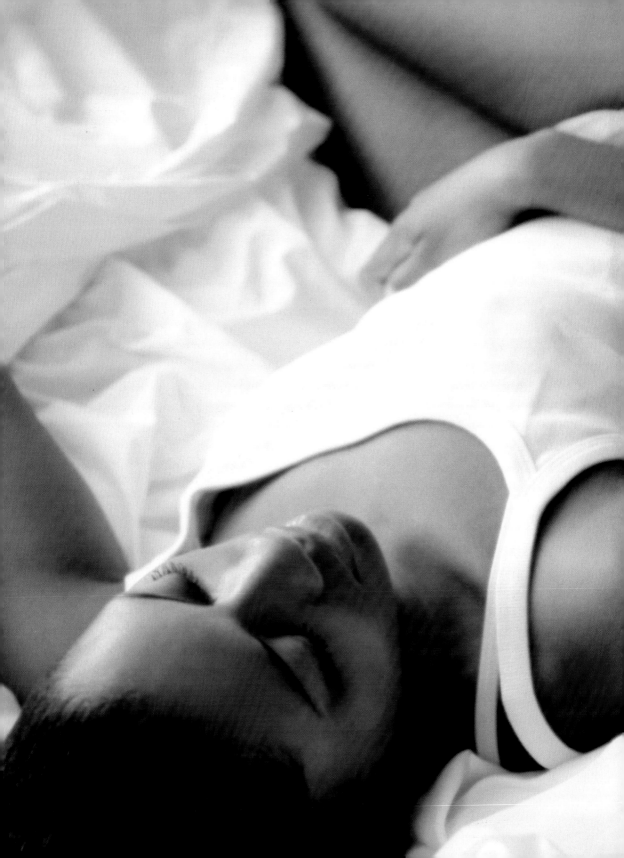

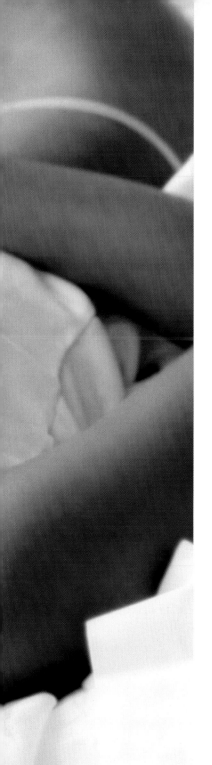

Best Advice From Black Doctors on Our Top 6 Health Concerns

The good news: If we do a better job of eating right, exercising and steering clear of toxins like cigarettes and too much alcohol, we can avoid potentially debilitating health conditions—or manage to live fulfilling lives in spite of them. Here's what you need to know about the top health challenges facing us, and the best advice from Black doctors on how to prevent and treat them. »

1. Heart Disease

What is heart disease?

It's a collective name for disorders that affect the heart's ability to function. This condition occurs when your arteries are blocked and oxygen and nutrients can't get to your heart.

Who gets it?

Heart disease is the number one killer of American women and men. For Black women, the incidence is particularly high: Heart disease kills more of us than AIDS, diabetes and cancer combined. Among women and men of all ethnicities, Black women also have the highest death rate. And we have an earlier onset: Most other groups of women experience heart trouble after menopause, but we tend to get heart disease in our forties.

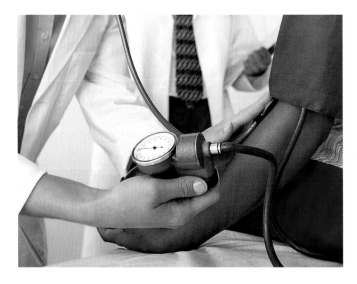

What does a heart attack feel like?

When we hear "heart attack," we often think of an older man clutching his chest, Fred Sanford-style. Although chest pain and heavy sweating are classic signs of a ticker in trouble, research shows that women are more likely than men to experience these unusual symptoms: persistent fatigue; pain right below the ribs or in the arms, neck or jaw; dizziness or nausea; shortness of breath; a burning sensation or sudden pressure in a seemingly unrelated area, such as the back.

Why are we affected more severely?

We tend to have a greater number of risk factors, such as obesity, smoking, high cholesterol, hypertension, type 2 diabetes and a family history of heart disease. Increasing age also plays a role. If you have one or more of these risk factors, let your doctor know and ask for the proper tests. Studies have shown that African-Americans don't undergo the same care for heart disease as Whites because they don't get the same tests and treatments, says Carlos S. Ince, M.D., a cardiologist at St. Agnes Hospital and Mid-Atlantic Cardiovascular in Baltimore and president of the Association of Black Cardiologists.

Prevention Prescription
7 Ways to Lower Your Heart Disease Risk

1. Quit smoking: Smoking destroys the protective lining of your arteries and is the biggest risk factor for sudden cardiac death. Talk to your doctor about nicotine-replacement products that may help you quit, and check out smokefree.gov for tips and resources.

2. Lower your blood pressure: Hypertension increases the heart's workload, causing its artery walls to stiffen, enlarging the heart and making it weaker. If your blood pressure exceeds 135/75, then it's too high. Cut salt from your diet; it can cause you to retain water, increasing blood pressure. Use other seasonings like herbs to make your food tasty.

3. Shed pounds: Excess weight puts an added strain on your heart. Losing just 10 percent of your weight can decrease your blood pressure.

4. Lower your cholesterol: Some of the foods we love don't love our body back. Fried indulgences are high in fat and cholesterol. Guidelines recommend an LDL (also known as the "bad" cholesterol) of below 130 mg/dL for those with moderate risk of heart disease. But health officials recently lowered LDL goals for those at very high risk, such as heart patients and diabetics, to under 70 mg/dL. Keep track of your numbers, and if they're too high, talk to your doctor about how to get them under control.

5. Study your family tree: Find out if heart disease runs in your family. Share that with your doctor, who can help you map out preventive strategies now.

6. Analyze your mood: Experts have tied depression, anger and even social isolation to an increased risk of heart disease. For your heart's sake, seek counseling if you need it and participate in activities that promote solid social relationships and help you relax (like prayer, yoga or meditation).

7. Build in more activity: Regular exercise helps increase blood flow to your heart, strengthening contractions and making it pump more efficiently. Physical activity also lowers your risk for other conditions that may tax your heart, including high blood pressure, high cholesterol and diabetes. Aim for 30 to 60 minutes of moderately intense activity four to six days per week. Walking, gardening, and taking the stairs all count toward your daily exercise quota.

Ask Yourself...

SHOULD I TAKE STATINS?

Statins seem to be the wonder drug: They drive down LDL cholesterol, reduce inflammation and stabilize the plaque that can clog your arteries. But not everyone needs them. Experts say you should consider statins if you fall into high-risk groups such as type 2 diabetics, patients who've already had a heart attack or people with moderate cholesterol levels and other risk factors such as smoking or hypertension. *Don't* take them if you're pregnant or breast-feeding, have chronic liver disease or are allergic to them.

WHAT IF I HAVE DIABETES?

Women with type 2 diabetes must also pay extra attention to their heart. Nearly three quarters of all diabetics die from cardiovascular problems, but there's an important distinction: Diabetic men have a 1.7 times higher risk of heart disease, while diabetic women have three times the risk.

SHOULD I HAVE AN ANEMIA TEST?

The Women's Ischemia Syndrome Evaluation (WISE) report noted that participants with anemia were more likely to have a heart attack, stroke or heart failure, and were almost twice as likely to die of heart disease. Anemia, a shortage of red blood cells, could make existing heart trouble more troublesome because it reduces the delivery of oxygen to the organs. In fact, anemia was a stronger predictor of serious heart disease than other risk factors, so get an anemia test during your yearly physical.

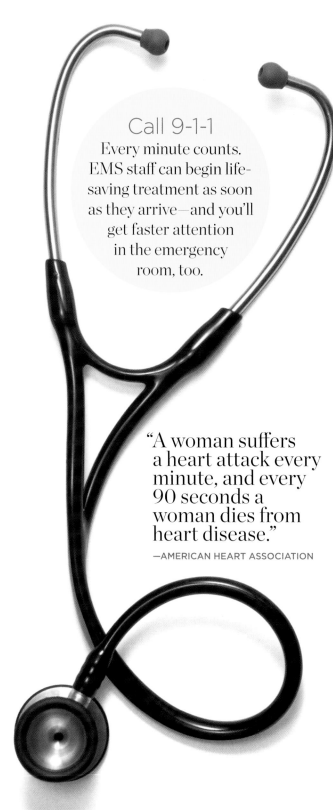

Call 9-1-1

Every minute counts. EMS staff can begin life-saving treatment as soon as they arrive—and you'll get faster attention in the emergency room, too.

"A woman suffers a heart attack every minute, and every 90 seconds a woman dies from heart disease."

—AMERICAN HEART ASSOCIATION

Experts long believed that estrogen made women less vulnerable than men to heart disease. Men were the priority for research, treatment and prevention efforts, and as a result doctors have mainly worked from a male-centered, one-size-fits-all model of the illness. But research from the Women's Ischemia Syndrome Evaluation (WISE) study—an analysis of nearly 1,000 female heart patients since 1996—found not only that women's symptoms can be more subtle and easier to ignore than men's, but also that the routine screenings our doctors rely on aren't always the best way to detect heart disease in women.

The **electrocardiogram (ECG) stress test**, which measures the electrical activity of your heart as you walk on a treadmill, is one of the most widely used screenings for heart disease. But while the ECG is 70 to 75 percent accurate in men, it works only 61 percent of the time for women. Researchers suspect that estrogen and progesterone, women's hormones, distort the results.

What's better for women is a combination of the **stress test and a CT scan or angiography**, says cardiologist Carlos Ince. With angiography, your doctor injects a dye into the artery of an arm or a leg, which allows her to see blockages. With the CT scan, the doctor takes a 3-D picture of your heart to detect levels of plaque. "The tests together are considered better for everybody, but for women in particular because of the false positives with stress tests," Ince says. Because the CT exposes you to X-rays, tell your doctor if you might be pregnant.

Unfortunately, insurance plans seldom cover angiography or CT tests, Ince says. If your insurance does not cover these tests, ask your doctor for **a stress nuclear test or a stress echo test**. Both take pictures of the heart, are 80 to 90 percent accurate in diagnosing heart disease in women and are more likely to be covered by insurance.

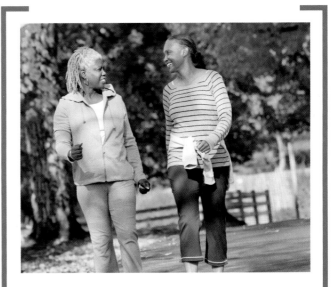

If You Do Just One Thing...

Move Your Body. Physical inactivity is a major risk factor for heart disease. Walk with a friend for a minimum of 20 to 30 minutes at least three times a week.

2. Stroke

What is stroke?

It is a blockage or rupture of a blood vessel that stops blood flow to the brain. Experts call stroke a "brain attack" because it is like a heart attack, but the damage occurs in your head.

Who's likely to have one?

Stroke is more prevalent among Black women than women in any other group. Black men and women have almost twice the risk of first-time strokes compared with Whites, and we have a higher death rate compared with Whites. While more men than women experience stroke, more women are likely to die from it. The key to surviving and recovering from a stroke is getting the right treatment in time.

What does a stroke feel like?

Sudden confusion, trouble speaking and understanding what others are saying, blurry vision, weakness, numbness or pain on one or both sides of your body. "The key word is 'sudden,'" says Gwendolyn F. Lynch, M.D., a stroke specialist at the Cleveland Clinic Foundation. "You should assume you're having a stroke until proven otherwise." Before having a full-blown stroke, some people have what's called a transient ischemic attack (TIA), in which the brain lacks oxygen for a brief period of time. A TIA is often described as a mini stroke; it is always an ominous sign that a stroke is coming. Symptoms of TIA, which are the same as those for stroke, last from 10 minutes to 24 hours, then disappear.

FAST Thinking

To get help quickly, the National Stroke Association encourages you to think FAST.

Face—Try to smile. Does one side of the face droop?
Arms—Raise both arms. Does one drift downward?
Speech–Try to say a simple sentence. Does it sound slurred?
Time –If you answer yes to any of these questions, call 911. Don't try to drive yourself to the hospital. A call to EMS gets you immediate attention and assures that you'll arrive in an ambulance, which can get you faster care.

Why are we affected more severely?

Risk factors such as hypertension, obesity, high cholesterol, type 2 diabetes, sickle cell anemia and a family history of stroke are more common in our families. Increasing age is also a factor, though younger African-American stroke victims die at higher rates than Whites in the same age group. Birth control pills and pregnancy, which can cause an increase in blood pressure, and using hormone therapy for menopause can raise your risks as well. Excessive alcohol and smoking are significant factors, too.

Prevention Prescription
6 ways to Decrease Your Risk of Stroke

1. Control your blood pressure: Hypertension is the number one risk factor for stroke. If your pressure exceeds 135/75, it's too high. Monitor birth control meds and cut salt from your diet. Both can cause an increase in blood pressure.

2. Stop smoking: Heavy cigarette smoking practically doubles your risk for stroke compared with light smokers. Better yet, quit altogether. Talk to your doctor about nicotine-replacement products, or check out smokefree.gov for tips.

3. Drink moderately: Alcohol can interact with your meds, and is also harmful in large quantities. Excessive drinking (more than one drink a day for women) has been tied to cancer, heart disease, liver disease and stroke.

4. Maintain a healthy weight: Exercise for 30 minutes at least three times a week, and avoid fatty foods.

5. Speak up: Ask your doctor to check circulation problems, which could mean that plaque is blocking your arteries. Tell your doctor if a relative has had a stroke.

6. Have your glucose levels tested: Get screened for diabetes by the time you're 45; earlier if you're at risk.

Don't Sleep on the Signs

At the first symptom of stroke, think of getting treatment as a race against the clock. If you delay, you may miss a critical window of time to receive drugs like the blood-clot-busting Tissue Plasminogen Activator (tPA), says Patrick A. Griffith, M.D., chair of neurology at Meharry Medical College in Nashville. "If you wait more than three hours, you're no longer a candidate," he says. "You lose the opportunity for brain damage to be reversible and fixable."

3. Cancer

What is cancer?

Cancer occurs when abnormal cells in a part of the body begin to grow out of control. Cancer cells outgrow normal cells and divide, spreading, or metastasizing, into other areas of the body. Cancer cells develop because of damage to your DNA. You can inherit damaged DNA through mutations in genes that normally protect against breast and ovarian cancer, such as BRCA1 or BRCA2 genes. Or your DNA can be damaged by environmental factors like chemicals, viruses (like HPV, which can lead to cervical cancer), tobacco smoke (which can lead to lung cancer) or too much sunlight (which can lead to skin cancer).

Who gets it?

Cancer is the second leading cause of death for African-American women. Half of all men and one third of all women in the United States will develop some form of cancer during their lifetimes. The leading types of cancer found in Black women are breast, lung and colon. Blacks have the highest death rate and the shortest survival rate of any racial group in the United States for most cancers.

What does having cancer feel like?

Different types of cancers act differently, depending on where they originate in the body. We explore the top three cancer threats—lung, breast and colon—in detail. Among other cancers, advanced cervical cancer sometimes causes vaginal discharge, vaginal pain during intercourse or bleeding after intercourse, while ovarian cancer, previously believed to be a silent disease, sometimes presents with a feeling of fullness in the pelvis, abdominal bloating or changes in bowel or bladder patterns.

Why are we affected more severely?

Our higher rate of obesity is a critical factor. Studies suggest one third of all cancer deaths are related to diet and obesity, which makes prevention the ultimate weapon in the war against the disease. Some forms of cancer are more aggressive in African-Americans, and we tend to seek treatment later than people of other races.

The Right Attention

If you or someone you know is diagnosed with cancer, insist that an oncology specialist be involved with treatment.

Prevention Prescription

What does it take to stay cancer-free? And what should you do once you're diagnosed? Here are 5 smart tips from African-American doctors that could save your life.

1. Figure out your risk: "If you have a family history of breast cancer, that's a red flag," says Lisa A. Newman, M.D., M.P.H., director at the University of Michigan Breast Care Center in Ann Arbor. Online tools can help you assess your risk. Two to try: Women's Cancer Network risk assessment survey for six types of female cancers (wcn.org) and National Cancer Institute (NCI) CARE Model risk assessment tool for breast cancer in African-American women (dceg.cancer.gov/tools/riskassessment/CARE).

2. Know the best defense: Eat right, which means increasing servings of cancer-fighting fruits and vegetables. Exercise is another must-do. Get your heart rate up for at least 30 minutes, three times a week. And don't smoke.

3. Don't be passive: "If cancer is more aggressive in Black women, then you have to be more aggressive in taking care of yourself," says B. Lee Green, Jr., Ph.D., vice-president of the Office of Institutional Diversity at the H. Lee Moffitt Cancer Center & Research Institute in Tampa. Be proactive when it comes to asking your doctor questions like: "How can I avoid getting breast cancer like my mom did?" "How accurate is this test?" "Why is this treatment best for me?"

4. Go with your gut: "Tell your doctor if something feels wrong," says Carol L. Brown, M.D., a gynecologic oncologist and associate attending surgeon at Memorial Sloan-Kettering Cancer Center in New York City. Some illnesses, such as breast cancer, are less likely to appear in young Black women, but symptoms can be more aggressive when they do, so timing is key.

5. Don't do it alone: If you're diagnosed with cancer, you may be too overwhelmed during doctor's appointments or too confused about how your health insurance works to look out for yourself. With a friend or family member by your side, you've got someone to help write down all your appointments and accompany you to treatments. You're also less likely to slip through the cracks of the health care system.

Black Women's Top Cancer Threats

CAN YOU GET CANCER FROM secondhand smoke? What are the signs of breast cancer? What foods can contribute to colon cancer? Experts reveal the answers and tell how to identify the top three cancers that afflict Black women.

Lung Cancer

WHO'S AT RISK: Smokers. Secondhand smoke, even at the club or a friend's house, can also put you at risk. In fact, secondhand smoke is responsible for about 3,400 lung cancer deaths annually among nonsmokers in the United States.

HOW TO DETECT IT: While there is no special screening for early detection of lung cancer, a recent study by the *New England Journal of Medicine* supports the idea that annual spiral CT scans could save the lives of smokers and former smokers by picking up lesions earlier. For now, those who exhibit symptoms should have a chest X-ray and a physical exam to check for lung abnormalities or swollen lymph nodes.

KNOW THE SIGNS:
* A persistent cough
* Chest pain
* Shortness of breath
* Chronic fatigue
* Headaches

Breast Cancer

WHO'S AT RISK: It can strike anyone, but some people stand a greater chance of developing the disease because of age (the majority of breast cancer patients are age 50 and older) and family history (you're more at risk if a close or distant relative has had the disease). Black women have a higher mortality rate from breast cancer than White women, although we're diagnosed with it less often. Scientists also know that Black women, especially those who are premenopausal, tend to get a type of breast cancer that is "high grade," or more aggressive, such as triple negative breast cancer.

HOW TO DETECT IT: Experts suggest regular clinical breast exams every three years for women in their twenties and thirties. Self-examinations done properly are also an option. Since the risk of breast cancer increases with age, women 40 and up should have annual mammograms. Women at a higher risk may need screenings earlier and more often. Depending on your risk, your doctor may have you supplement mammograms with MRIs, sonograms or digital mammograms (which can better examine dense breast tissue), or devise a preventive game plan for you.

KNOW THE SIGNS:

* A firm breast lump that isn't easily moved
* Spontaneous nipple discharge other than milk
* Change in texture of skin around the nipple
* Increase in breast size over a short time (maybe a cup size in a few days)
* Unrelenting itching
* Swollen lymph nodes in the underarm or above or below the collarbone

Colon Cancer

WHO'S AT RISK: Black women die of colon cancer at a rate more than 40 percent higher than White women. James A. Posey III, M.D., associate professor of medicine at the University of Alabama at Birmingham, cites "supersize" diets, lifestyle and inadequate health care as possible factors.

HOW TO DETECT IT: Starting at age 50, screen for colon cancer with a digital rectal exam every five years and a fecal occult blood test annually. Women should also have a colonoscopy. Higher-risk patients should be screened more frequently.

KNOW THE SIGNS:

* Occasional blood in the stool
* Sudden change in bowel habits
* Pencil-thin stool
* Unusual stomach pain
* Fatigue
* Unexplained weight loss

Ask Yourself...

WHO WILL UNDERSTAND? If you've been diagnosed with cancer, it might be helpful to find common ground in a support group. Within the circle of people who can relate to what you're experiencing, you can comfortably say things you might be afraid to say to your friends and family members. "Every day we link women to others in the community who have recently been successfully treated for some kind of cancer," says Karen E. Jackson, founder and CEO of Sisters Network, Inc., the country's only African-American breast cancer survivorship organization (sistersnetworkinc.org). The American Cancer Society also has a range of support groups all over the country.

Help find a cure...

Even if you're not a cancer patient, you can help with research. Participating in a clinical trial—which can be as simple as filling out a survey—helps doctors gather accurate data on how diseases and drugs affect different groups of people. Studies have shown that African-Americans are less likely than Whites to be involved in clinical trials, and sadly, that leads to lack of research specific to how drugs react in our bodies. To find out if you qualify for a clinical trial, cancer-free or not, visit Web sites like cancer.gov/clinicaltrials (a resource for more than 6,000 cancer clinical trials) and wcn.org (Women's Cancer Network). If you have cancer, talk to your primary care physician about joining a trial.

4. Obesity

What does it mean to be obese?

Obesity is a condition in which you have too much body weight for your height. Doctors determine body fat by using the Body Mass Index (BMI), a formula based on your weight and height. They also consider your waist measurement to be an indicator of appropriate weight (35 inches or more for women is too much). The more obese or overweight you are, the higher your risk for a number of conditions, including diabetes, heart disease and stroke, hypertension and some cancers.

Calculating Your BMI

You can figure out your Body Mass Index (BMI) by using the following formula or by entering your information in the calculator at cdc.gov/nccd/php/bmi/index.htm. BMI = weight (pounds) x 703 ÷ height (inches) squared

If you're number is:	You're considered:
less than 18.5	underweight
18.5 to 24.9	healthy
25 to 29	overweight
30 and above	obese

Who is obese or overweight?

Unfortunately, far too many of us: "The epidemic of obesity in America is growing, particularly among Black women," says Lynn Rosenberg, Sc.D., principal investigator of the Black Women's Health Study, one of the largest longitudinal studies conducted of African-American women's health. About two thirds of U.S. adults are obese or overweight, as are 61.6 percent of women. Among Black women, however, that figure soars to nearly 80 percent.

Why are our obesity rates so much higher?

Experts say obesity is a result of a number of factors, including your family history, high-calorie, high-fat diets, lack of access to fresh foods and limited physical activity. There are also cultural factors, says Nelson L. Adams, M.D., president of the National Medical Association and chair of the obstetrics and gynecology department at Jackson North Medical Center in Miami, Florida. "It is accepted in our community that full-figured is okay," Adams says. "We tend to feel less guilt about overeating. That perhaps dates to a historical time when there wasn't enough to eat." Whatever the factors, the bottom line is that more of us are overweight or obese because we consume more calories than our bodies burn through exercise.

Prevention Prescription
Experts take a closer look at the obesity epidemic and explain how we can stop it.

Q. Many people chalk up being overweight to genetics. How much of a role does family history play?

A. "There's always been the notion of genetics versus the environment," Adams says. "If you look at some families, people say, 'If Grandma is heavy, I'm going to be heavy.' But that doesn't mean you will be obese; you're just more likely to put on weight. The doubling of our children's rates of obesity is more than genetic."

Q. How does where we live affect our weight?

A. "In many neighborhoods, we lack access to fresh fruits and vegetables," says Janice Whitty, M.D., director of maternal fetal medicine at Meharry Medical College in Nashville. "Or it's so expensive that junk food ends up being cheaper than a healthy diet. And in many cities and towns, we no longer have sidewalks. People don't walk anymore; we drive everywhere."

Q. If obesity is "epidemic," why aren't we more alarmed?

A. "What's happened is that we have adjusted to new, bigger sizes—even doctors," Whitty says. "We've seen so many people large for so long that our eyes are adjusting to larger bodies. If I don't calculate the BMI, I won't realize that a patient is overweight."

Q. What's the best first step to losing weight?

A. "Start with very practical, easy things to do, and aim for small successes," Adams says. Cut back on alcohol; it's just calories without the nutrients. Trim the bread from your diet. "No corn bread, no biscuits," Adams says. Get yourself a pedometer and aim for 10,000 steps a day, about 5 miles. If you take the stairs instead of the escalator, those steps add up quick.

Ask Yourself...

WHY LOSE?

You probably know the benefits of losing weight: healthier heart, lower cholesterol, reduced risks of diseases. But here are some that might surprise you:

A good night's sleep Weight loss can improve sleep apnea, a condition in which you stop breathing for short periods during the night.

Greater flexibility Losing 5 percent of your weight reduces stress on your knees, hips and lower back, and lessens your risk for osteoarthritis.

An easier pregnancy You'll lower your risk of gestational diabetes and preeclampsia and be less likely to need a cesarean delivery.

Hotter sex With a boosted body image, you'll set off sparks between the sheets.

5. Diabetes

What is diabetes?

Diabetes occurs when your body does not use insulin properly. Your body needs insulin to convert the sugars in food into energy. With type 1 diabetes (typically first diagnosed in children or young adults), the body destroys the cells in the pancreas that make insulin. With type 2, the body either can't produce enough insulin or it becomes resistant to the insulin produced. With gestational diabetes, which develops in about 1 in 20 women during pregnancy, the body produces more of certain hormones that make it resistant to insulin.

Who gets it?

More than 13 percent of African-Americans 20 or older—about 3.2 million—have diabetes, and one in four Black women over 55 has it. Diabetes is the fourth leading cause of death for Black men and women.

What does having diabetes feel like?

The symptoms can be so subtle that one third of all people with diabetes don't even know they have it. Symptoms may include unusual thirst, frequent urination, extreme hunger, weight loss, blurred vision, weakness and fatigue, irritability and mood changes, nausea and vomiting. Type 2 is also characterized by frequent infections that heal slowly; dry, itchy skin; and tingling or loss of feeling in the hands or feet.

What are the risks of developing diabetes?

For type 1, the only risk factor is family history. Factors contributing to type 2 also include ethnicity, increased age, excess weight, physical inactivity, high blood pressure, abnormal cholesterol, a history of gestational diabetes and giving birth to a baby weighing more than nine pounds.

What tests will tell me if I have diabetes?

Several doctor-administered blood tests detect the disease: a Fasting Plasma Glucose Test measures the amount of sugar in your blood after you have refrained from eating or drinking for eight hours; a Random Plasma Glucose Test measures your blood sugar at any given time; and an Oral Glucose Tolerance Test first measures your fasting blood sugar, then tests your blood sugar at intervals for two to three hours after you drink a sugary solution.

What's prediabetes?

It's a condition more than 50 million Americans have; your blood sugar levels are high, but not at the level of diabetes. Prediabetics have a greater than 50 percent chance of developing diabetes over the next ten years, and a 50 percent higher risk of heart attack or stroke than people with normal blood glucose levels. Unlike diabetes, prediabetes may be reversible.

Prevention Prescription
5 Ways to Lower Your Diabetes Risks

1. Get your glucose levels tested: Make sure you get screened by age 45; earlier if you're at risk.

2. Eat right: Follow a low-fat, reduced-calorie diet, as excess weight can increase your chances of getting diabetes. Opt for leafy green vegetables and whole grains. Drink plenty of water. Bake or broil meat, chicken and fish. If you're prediabetic, see a nutritionist.

3. Find time to unwind: An increase in stress can translate to an increase in blood glucose levels. Even if it's ten minutes a day, relax and enjoy a hot bath, listen to soothing music or meditate.

4. Get physical: Walking for 30 minutes five days a week can tame tension and get you on the road to slimming down.

5. Ask your doctor about medication: Diet and exercise changes have been shown to be more effective than oral drugs like metformin. But if your glucose levels show that you're prediabetic and you have a serious family history of diabetes, you may want to discuss drugs as a second-tier approach with your doctor.

Ask Yourself...

WHAT'S "DIABESITY?"

It's a new term that seeks to describe the close relationship between diabetes and obesity. Diabesity refers to the trend of adult obesity being accompanied by diabetes. "Diabetes follows obesity almost like a shadow," says Valentine J. Burroughs, M.D., M.B.A., senior vice-president of medical affairs at Saint Francis Hospital in Wilmington, Delaware. "Being overweight or obese can lead to insulin resistance."

A Winning Strategy

"People with prediabetes can often prevent or delay developing diabetes by losing about 7 percent of their body weight," says Griffin P. Rodgers, M.D., director of the National Institute of Diabetes and Digestive and Kidney Diseases at the National Institutes of Health.

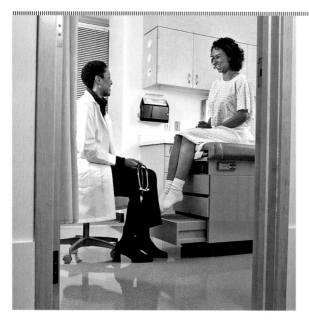

Ask the Docs About Diabetes

Does having diabetes mean I have to take insulin? If you have type 1 diabetes, yes. Because your pancreas produces little or no insulin, the hormone has to be injected. With type 2 diabetes, you can start with oral medications, then follow up with insulin if the diabetes isn't controlled, says Wilma J. Wooten, M.D., M.P.H., principal investigator for the National Medical Association's diabetes education program. Amaryl and Glucophage are two oral medications that address how glucose is used in your body.

Does getting diabetes mean I'll die soon? "Absolutely not," says Valentine J. Burroughs, M.D., M.B.A., senior vice-president of medical affairs at Saint Francis Hospital in Wilmington, Delaware. "If it's managed properly, there is no reason for your life to be any shorter than a person without diabetes." However, about 65 percent of African-American diabetics who die do so from heart disease or stroke. And nerve damage affects millions of diabetics, putting them at risk for foot injury, infection and even amputation. Eating whole, nonprocessed foods and controlling your weight are key to avoiding complications. So is reducing stress. "A lot of chronic illnesses are brought on by tension and depression," explains Burroughs.

Does having diabetes mean I'll go blind? Diabetics are 60 percent more likely to develop cataracts, and diabetes is the leading cause of new cases of blindness among adults ages 20 to 74. But it helps to be vigilant. "During the eye exam, you can detect changes or abnormalities in retinal tissue. If addressed early, the visual prognosis is better," says Derrick L. Artis, O.D., M.B.A., an optometrist and vice-president of Vision Source. Artis recommends a dilated retinal exam once a year for patients with the condition.

Can I ever get off my meds? Possibly. "If you have type 2 diabetes," says Wooten, "you can reduce the need for or the amount of medication, depending on how severe the condition is, if you lose weight." In obese people, Wooten says, fat cells cover the receptors for insulin and make it impossible for the body to process glucose. If you're prediabetic, she says, "you can definitely stave off the onset of diabetes by losing just 5 to 7 percent of your total body weight." If you have type 1 diabetes, meaning your pancreas has stopped producing insulin, you will have to take meds to make up for what the pancreas doesn't produce.

6. HIV

What is HIV?

The acronym stands for Human Immunodeficiency Virus, which is the virus that causes AIDS. It may be spread through infected blood or unprotected sexual contact. Infected women also can pass HIV to their babies through pregnancy or delivery—although there are drugs to prevent this—and through breast-feeding.

What is AIDS?

Acquired Immunodeficiency Syndrome, or AIDS, occurs when HIV weakens the immune system and certain infections or cancers develop. A decrease in a person's immune cells is also a sign of AIDS.

Who gets HIV/AIDS?

Although Blacks make up 13 percent of the population, they accounted for half of the new HIV/AIDS diagnoses in the United States from 2001 to 2004, according to the Centers for Disease Control. Black men make up nearly 44 percent of new diagnoses among men, while Black women represent an astounding 67 percent of cases diagnosed among women.

Why are we affected more severely?

Studies have linked AIDS cases to the problems connected with poverty, including lack of quality health care and adequate housing, as well as lack of HIV awareness and prevention education. But high-risk sexual contact (with men who have multiple partners, men who sleep with men or men who are IV drug users) is the most frequent method of transmission for Black women (74 percent) followed by intravenous drug use (24 percent).

Our Top Risk Factor

Twenty years ago, the face of HIV/AIDS was that of a gay White male. In 2008, that face is more likely to look like us. HIV/AIDS is the leading cause of death for Black women ages 25 to 35, the third leading cause for those ages 35 to 44 and the fourth leading cause for those ages 45 to 54.How did we get here? "Most often the significant risk factor for Black women is the fact that they've had unprotected sex with the wrong man," says Valerie E. Stone, M.D., M.P.H., director of the Women's HIV/AIDS Program at Massachusetts General Hospital in Boston and associate professor of medicine at Harvard.

5 reasons why the rate of HIV/AIDS diagnoses among Black women is higher than that of any other group:

1 MULTIPLE SEX PARTNERS. When both partners are having sex outside the relationship, says Adaora Adimora, M.D., M.P.H., associate professor of medicine at the University of North Carolina, you can see HIV/AIDS worming its way through our community "like a tree branching."

2 HIGHER RATES OF SEXUALLY TRANSMITTED INFECTIONS. In 2005, Blacks were 18 times more likely than Whites to have gonorrhea and 5 times more likely to have syphilis. Certain STIs can increase your risk of contracting HIV.

3 DRUG USE. Injecting drugs is the second leading cause of HIV infection for Black women and men. Illegal drug users are also more likely to take risks, like having unprotected sex while high.

4 HIGHER RATES OF POVERTY. Poverty destabilizes many relationships, and people living in poverty are more likely to come into contact with someone at risk for HIV. "But don't think you're immune because you're not poor," Adimora says.

5 DENIAL AND STIGMA. They keep us from recognizing our degree of risk, from using condoms and from getting tested. "Women don't ask to get tested because they're worried about what people think of them," says HIV/AIDS expert Valerie E. Stone. Our fears also keep us from talking about homosexuality, drug use, concurrent sexual practices and other factors that put us at greater risk.

Make Testing Routine

Twenty-five percent of people with HIV don't know they have the virus. The Centers for Disease Control and Prevention recommend that HIV screening be a routine part of medical care for adults and adolescents. "Black people tend to die more often than Whites and Latinos from HIV-related complications because testing is often done late in the course of the disease, making it more difficult to treat," says David J. Malebranche, M.D., M.P.H., assistant professor of general medicine at Emory University. Adds Valerie Stone: "Ideally the HIV test will become as routine as a Pap smear."

Emergency HIV Intervention: Postexposure prophylaxis, or PEP, is a 28-day treatment that may reduce your chances of HIV infection by up to 81% when taken within 72 hours of exposure. Call your doctor or local AIDS organizations.

Prevention Prescription
How to protect yourself from HIV/AIDS

1. Abstain from sex: That includes not having oral, vaginal and anal sex until you are in a relationship with only one person, are having sex only with each other, and you each know the other's HIV status. "Get tested together before you stop using condoms," Stone suggests.

2. Use a latex lubricated condom: Open up that condom packet every time you have sex. "Discuss it before your clothes are off, otherwise you will risk anger and disappointment," Stone says.

3. Get tested: Whenever you have a medical checkup, or if you are planning to get pregnant or are pregnant, get screened for HIV.

4. Be up-front: If you have multiple partners, talk about HIV and other STIs with each partner before you have sex.

5. Be vigilant: If you think you may have been exposed, get tested and also get treated for other STIs.

6. Just say no: Don't inject illegal drugs. And don't have sex when you are taking drugs or drinking alcohol; being high can make you more likely to take risks.

HIV Q&A
We tackle some common questions and little-known facts about the virus.

....

Q **Can women give men HIV?**
A It's true that it is harder for men to get HIV from women—men have fewer areas on the penis where the virus can enter the bloodstream (such as the opening of the tip or through cuts or sores on the shaft). But if either partner has an STI, especially one with lesions, his risk greatly increases.

Q **How does having an STI increase the risk for HIV/AIDS?**
A Because of inflammation and an increase in white blood cells, STIs (especially those that cause lesions) can make it easier for HIV to enter the bloodstream. STIs like gonorrhea can also increase the amount of HIV, or "viral load," in semen.

Q **I've heard of the HIV Rapid Test. How does that work?**
A To find a free or low-cost clinic in your area, visit hivtest.org and enter your zip code. Some locations offer anonymous testing. You'll receive precounseling to review the risk factors and answer your questions. You'll either get a finger prick or an oral swab along your gum line. After the specimen is collected, it takes about 20 minutes to get results. If the results are negative, the counselor will talk with you about lowering your risk. If positive, you'll take a second test to confirm, then discuss health care providers and what help you'll need.

Medical Tests to Get at Every Age

Your 20s

- Pap test and pelvic exam annually, including a screening for sexually transmitted infections (STIs); more often if you have multiple sex partners, are HIV-positive or have a weakened immune system
- An in-office breast exam
- Blood-pressure test
- Cholesterol test
- Blood glucose–diabetes test
- Dental exams twice yearly
- A complete eye exam every two years; annually if you wear glasses or contact lenses. If anyone in your family has glaucoma, make sure an ophthalmologist performs a visual field test and checks your eye pressure
- A skin exam

Your 30s

- Pap test and pelvic exam annually, including a screening for sexually transmitted infections (STIs); more often if you have multiple sex partners, are HIV-positive or have a weakened immune system
- Clinical breast exam
- Baseline mammogram at age 35 if you have a family history of breast cancer (otherwise at 40)
- Blood-pressure test
- Cholesterol test
- Blood glucose–diabetes test
- Thyroid test (TSH) at age 35, then once every five years
- A complete eye exam every two years; annually if you wear glasses or contacts
- Dental exams twice yearly
- Skin exam

Keep this checklist handy to make sure you get the proper health screenings at your annual checkup. Your doctor may suggest additional tests depending on your medical profile, which should include your family's health history. As a general rule, here are the tests that you'll need. >>

Your 40s

- ☐ Pap test and pelvic exam annually, including a screening for sexually transmitted infections (STIs); more often if you have multiple sex partners, are HIV-positive or have a weakened immune system
- ☐ Mammogram
- ☐ Blood-pressure test
- ☐ Cholesterol test
- ☐ Thyroid test (TSH)
- ☐ Blood glucose–diabetes test
- ☐ Obesity screening
- ☐ Bone-mineral and bone-mass measurement at age 40 if you have a predisposition for osteoporosis due to medication, or have a disease associated with bone loss
- ☐ A complete eye exam every two years; annually if you wear glasses or contacts
- ☐ Glaucoma screening
- ☐ Dental exams twice yearly
- ☐ A skin exam

Your 50s

- ☐ Pap test and pelvic exam annually, including a screening for sexually transmitted infections (STIs); more often if you have multiple sex partners, are HIV-positive or have a weakened immune system
- ☐ Mammogram
- ☐ Blood-pressure test
- ☐ Cholesterol test
- ☐ Colonoscopy
- ☐ Bone density test
- ☐ Blood glucose–diabetes test
- ☐ Obesity screening
- ☐ Thyroid test (TSH) once every five years
- ☐ A complete eye exam every two years; annually if you wear glasses or contacts
- ☐ Glaucoma screening
- ☐ Dental exams twice yearly
- ☐ Auditory screening
- ☐ A skin exam

Cover Yourself: Health Insurance Strategies

If you're among the one in three African-American women with no health insurance, don't let fear or lack of knowledge stand in the way of your health care. Take the time to do a thorough search for sources of individual health insurance—coverage you pay for outright that isn't connected to an employer. Here's how to start:

Check out organizations. **Many advocacy, alumni, professional, religious and trade associations have negotiated discounts with insurance companies, says health educator David Nganele, Ph.D. "By becoming a member you can get lower-cost group coverage."**

Keep COBRA. **A federal law, COBRA allows you to keep your employee health benefits for up to 18 months after leaving a job. Once your 18 months are up, HIPAA, another federal law, lets you buy an individual policy through the same insurer.**

Go independent. **If you need to buy an individual policy, consult a knowledgeable independent agent. She'll explain the ratings process and help you comparison-shop for the best value.**

Open a Health Savings Account. **An HSA combines a high-deductible policy with a tax-sheltered savings account. Basically, you sign up for a policy that covers large hospital bills. Once you've met the insurer's deductible, you're free to withdraw funds from the savings account to pay medical expenses. What you don't spend collects interest. (For a guide to setting up an HSA, go to hsainsider.com.)**

Check with the state. **Many states offer coverage for low-income residents who have been deemed uninsurable because they suffer from chronic diseases. The catch: Many have long waiting lists and stringent income requirements. Call the insurance board in your state.**

Understand the lingo. **Healthinsuranceinfo.net, which is maintained by Georgetown University's Health Policy Institute, offers state-by-state guides and a glossary of terms; and *Making Them Pay: How to Get the Most From Health Insurance and Managed Care* by Rhonda D. Orin (St. Martin's Griffin), shows you how to read and understand a health plan.**

Your Wellness Goals

What are your top three health concerns?
Note anything from a hereditary disease you want to prevent to embarrassing questions, such as bladder-control problems.

1 _____
2 _____
3 _____

What health issues have you or a relative had since your last doctor visit?

_____
_____

Have you noticed any changes in how your body feels or functions?

Vision _____
Breasts _____
Weight _____
Urinary/bowel habits _____
Skin _____
Menstrual cycle _____
Emotions _____

What hurts right now?

_____
_____

Appointment checklist:
Note date and time of your next exam

☐ Primary-care doctor _____
☐ Ob-gyn _____
☐ Optometrist _____
☐ Dentist _____
☐ Specialists _____

Don't Forget to Ask Your Doctor...

What's my risk for heart disease?
What's my blood pressure? What does it mean for me and what do I need to do?
What are my cholesterol levels (LDL, HDL and triglycerides)? What do they mean for me, and what do I need to do about them?
What's my body mass index (BMI) and waist measurement? Do they mean I need to lose weight for my health?
What is my blood sugar level, and does it mean that I'm at risk for diabetes? If so, what should I do about it?
Based on my history and your observations, what other screenings or tests do I need?
Can I be tested for HIV/AIDS?

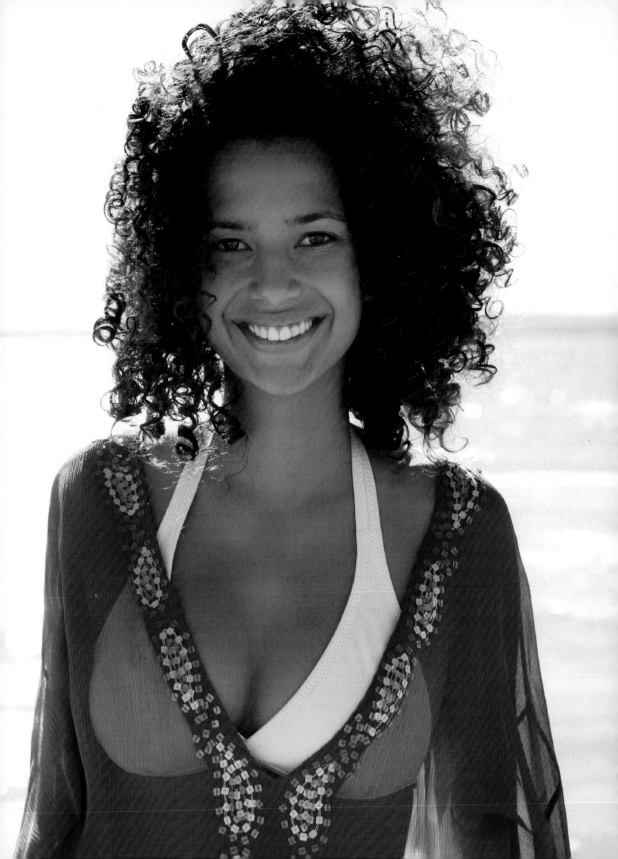

Part 2: Fit + Fabulous

You Can Do It! }

As Black women, we embrace our curves. In fact, according to an Indiana University study, African-American women continue to have a more favorable body image than White women. But let's get real: Being overweight contributes to and complicates serious medical problems from diabetes and heart disease to some cancers. That's why it's critical that we not only maintain a healthy weight, but also stay active to keep our heart healthy and our muscles strong. Whether you need to lose 10 pounds or more than 100, we'll show you how to set realistic goals for consistent progress and bring you the latest wisdom from leading experts. For your workout, we give you exercise moves that will firm you up all over, improve your mood, help you get a better night's sleep and possibly even boost your sex life. We even offer solutions to common challenges that keep you from embracing healthier diet and exercise habits (does "I don't want to sweat out my hair!" sound familiar?). Ready? Let's go! »

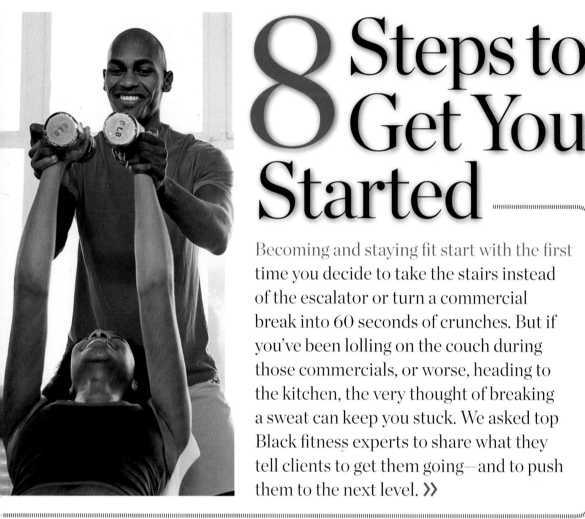

8 Steps to Get You Started

Becoming and staying fit start with the first time you decide to take the stairs instead of the escalator or turn a commercial break into 60 seconds of crunches. But if you've been lolling on the couch during those commercials, or worse, heading to the kitchen, the very thought of breaking a sweat can keep you stuck. We asked top Black fitness experts to share what they tell clients to get them going—and to push them to the next level. »

1 Come As You Are

COMMITTING TO A FITNESS ROUTINE means tuning in to your love and respect for your body, says celebrity trainer Kacy Duke, author of *The Show It Love Workout* (McGraw-Hill). Before you do even one leg lift, she says, practice accepting yourself just as you are. Then get clear about what you want to make even better. Here's how: ✳ Take a good look at your body in front of a mirror or have a friend or trainer help you assess yourself in a bathing suit. Use this feedback to develop your workout goals. ✳ Promise your body that you'll honor and respect it every day. ✳ Come up with ways to address the issues that keep you stuck (you might need a therapist to help you deal with some of these). ✳ "Once you've built this foundation," Duke says, "tell yourself, 'This is where I am right now, but now I need more.'"

2
Find Your Motivation

KNOW WHY YOU WANT AND NEED to exercise—not why you *should*, says Dallas R. Fuentes, a certified Pilates instructor and owner-director of Perfect Parts Pilates, Inc., in New York City. What's likely to keep you going is recognizing what truly motivates you. There are no right or wrong reasons, so examine what matters to you and check all that apply.

- ☐ to improve my health
- ☐ to like what I see in the mirror
- ☐ to feel better
- ☐ to be stronger
- ☐ to fit into my favorite jeans
- ☐ for better sex

- ☐ to be more attractive
- ☐ to compete in a sport
- ☐ to keep up with my kids
- ☐ so my knees/back/neck/feet won't hurt

- ☐ because I don't want to go up another size
- ☐ to feel good about myself
- ☐ _____ _____ (fill in your own reason)

3
Imagine You, Only Better

PICTURE WHAT YOU WANT your body to look like, Fuentes says. But don't base that picture on some other person's body. "Nothing's more beautiful on you than what you have," she says. Keeping your ideal image in mind, identify the areas you want to work on. Your overall goal could be to shed pounds, but you may also want to target your waist or tone your arms. This is the basis of your exercise plan.

How Fast Can I Slim Down?

Think those "Drop 5 pounds in 5 days" ads are realistic? Consider this: **You've got to burn about 3,500 calories to lose a pound.** It takes about 45 minutes to an hour of aerobics and stretching to burn between 300 and 600 calories, says trainer Aisha Cowart. To zap 3,500 calories in a day, you'd have to exercise for nearly six hours and not eat at all. A healthier and more realistic goal is to lose a pound or two each week.

Find Your Target Heart Rate

Everybody says "boost your heart rate to burn calories," but how much is enough? It depends on your age, says New Jersey-based trainer and fitness consultant Benita Perkins. To measure your heart rate, or your pulse, place your middle two fingers on the side of your neck, just under your jawbone. Count the number of beats in ten seconds, and multiply that number by six. Adjust your workout accordingly. If you can't measure your pulse, a general rule is that you should be able to carry on a conversation while working out, suggests the American Heart Association (AHA). If you're too winded, slow your pace. If your talk seems too easy, step it up.

Target Heart Rate Zone by Age	
20s	98–170 beats per minute
30s	93–162 beats per minute
40s	88–153 beats per minute
50s	83–145 beats per minute

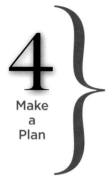

Make a Plan

IF YOU KNOW YOUR GOAL, YOU'LL HAVE A BETTER IDEA OF HOW TO ATTAIN IT

GOAL	BEST EXERCISE	WHAT IT DOES	HOW TO GET IT
"Better health." "Because I've always wanted to run a 10k."	Cardio/aerobics	Boosts heart rate, improves lung capacity and endurance	Walking briskly, jogging/running, circuit training, spinning, biking
"To look better in that black dress." "To tone and firm."	Resistance training, weight training	Strengthens muscles	Lifting weights, squats, lunges, resistance bands, biking, swimming
"So my knees won't hurt." "To increase strength."	Supervised weight training	Strengthens bones	Lifting weights, circuit training
"To feel better." "To have greater flexibility and posture."	Stretching, bending, flexing	Stretches and lengthens muscles	Yoga, Pilates, tai chi

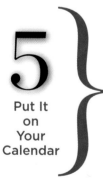

Put It on Your Calendar

MAKE TIME FOR YOURSELF. "Schedule your workout in your date book just like anything else," Fuentes says. No time? Take a look at your schedule and see what you can let go. "Instead of getting your nails done, you could be home stretching," she says. Instead of grabbing the chips and settling in for your favorite TV show, work out while you watch.

Healthy Returns—what you can buy if you skip that daily latte and invest in your fitness:

$15	An exercise book, video or DVD
$25	Free weights or dumbbells (a set of 3 lb, 5 lb or 8 lb); a stability ball
$100	A session with a trainer
$150	Another round with the trainer, plus some cute workout wear!

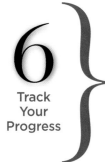

6
Track Your Progress

KEEP A JOURNAL. At least once a day, write down your goals and assess how you measured up. (You can start on page 148.) Don't get discouraged if your goals sometimes exceed your reach, Duke says. See it as a mark to aim for the next day. Soon enough, you'll be able to look back and see how far you've come. And if your plan gets stalled, you'll be able to see why and make corrections. Here's a sample entry:

> Sept. 14 What's Your Health Goal for the Day?: Dance 20 mins, stretch 10 mins Notes: Did I get there? Barely! My heart was pumping hard, but it felt good to be moving and not be out of breath. Can't believe that when I started, I could only dance for 5 minutes before getting winded. Think I'll add 3 minutes tomorrow!

7
Never Skip Meals

NOT EATING REGULARLY sends your body into starvation mode, says Aisha Cowart, director of personal training, nutrition and group conditioning at Eastern Athletic Clubs in New York. "The moment the body feels hungry it starts to store any food you put in it as fat." If you don't want to fool your brain into thinking that you're starving, eat at least three meals a day, with healthy snacks in between.

8
Get Your Zzz's

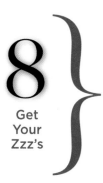

BELIEVE IT OR NOT, Cowart says, getting seven hours of sleep each night helps you continue burning calories: "If you're aerobic through the day," she says, "by the time your body goes to rest, it's able to metabolize properly through the night." On the other hand, not getting enough sleep puts your body in stress mode, causing it to burn calories more slowly.

Should You Consult a Trainer?

If you need an objective assessment of what kind of workout plan you need, you might want to enlist the services of a personal trainer. She or he will meet with you, get a health and fitness history and risk assessment, then work with you to clarify your goals and map out a strategy to reach them. When considering a trainer, keep in mind the four C's:

COST: Trainers set their own fees, which can range from $40 to $120-plus an hour.

CONVENIENCE: You may need a trainer who can come to your home at 6:00 A.M., or who can meet you at the gym right after work. A regular workout schedule is key.

CERTIFICATION: Credentials reflect a trainer's ability to consistently meet industry standards. Many agencies certify trainers, but three of the most reputable are the American Council on Exercise (ACE, 888-825-3636; acefitness.org), the National Academy of Sports Medicine (NASM, 800-460-6276; nasm.org), and the National Strength and Conditioning Association (NSCA, 800-815-6826; ncsa-lift.org). Contact them to verify trainer credentials.

COMPATIBILITY: A good trainer is attentive and focused on helping you reach your goals safely. You need to feel comfortable enough to be honest about everything from your weight to those extra scoops of ice cream you had. Ask yourself: "Is this someone I can trust?"

"I Lost With My Family"

Here's one sibling's story of how making a plan with her four sisters to lose weight together—445 pounds and counting!—was the key to her success.

AFTER
Williams at her goal weight and below with her sisters

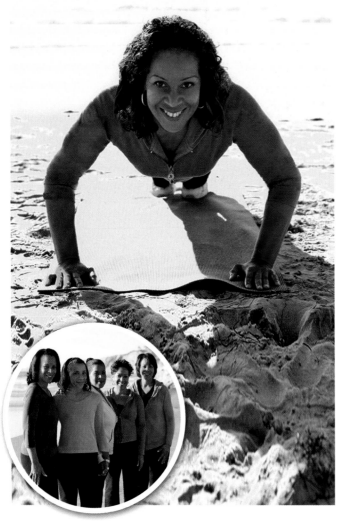

PAMELA WILLIAMS, 49
HEIGHT: 5′3″
BEFORE: 191 lbs
NOW: 135 lbs
WEIGHT LOSS: 56 lbs

"I was in total denial," says Pamela Williams, an administrative assistant in San Diego. Instead of admitting that her midsection was too plump, she would tell herself she was bloated. And for years Williams was also sabotaging her own weight-loss efforts. "I always exercised, but I'd go for a walk and then treat myself to a burger and some fries afterward, thinking that was all right," she says.

Then her sister DeJeanette stepped up to the Weight Watchers plate and started encouraging her other four sisters to do the same. When Pamela got onto a scale at the beginning of the program, she was served a dose of reality that brought tears to her eyes. But she became determined to bring her number down, adding strength training, ramping up her cardio routines and pedaling circles on her favorite machine: the elliptical trainer. She also booted some of her comfort-food habits, such as indulging in Mexican fare and cookies.

Her key to staying on track? "Everything in moderation," she says. "Now I can have one chocolate chip cookie and it's okay. Before I would eat seven or eight." Pamela's biggest victory? "Just knowing that I can go to my water aerobics class and not be embarrassed to take off my towel."

One of the biggest motivators was having her sisters to help keep her in line. The family still gathers for lightened-up Sunday dinners (that "fried" chicken is baked now), goes walking as a group and keeps track of one another's progress through phone calls. Plus, the sisters inspired their mom, Vera, 71, to join their healthy living crusade! Vera's lost 22 pounds so far; her goal is 25.

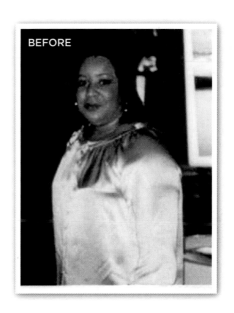

BEFORE

Expert's Advice: Get Your Group Going

As the Williams sisters know, a weight loss group can bolster your spirit and give you the support you need to become healthy. Rovenia Brock, Ph.D., author of *Dr. Ro's Ten Secrets to Livin' Healthy* (Bantam), suggests these tips for starting a group of your own:

1. **Invite people who are committed** to making a change and are already in your social circle: women you see at church, coworkers, other moms in the PTA. That way the members start off with a sense of comfort, cohesion and accountability to one another.

2. **Decide when everyone will meet.** Will it be Saturday morning for a workout with a trainer whose fee you all split? Twice a month for a healthy-recipe potluck dinner? When you do get together, talk about success strategies and let each person share.

3. **Establish goals and a plan to achieve them.** Do you want to lose a pound a week? Train for a 5K race? Look cute in a bikini? Figure out what you want to accomplish, then do research or seek the assistance of a nutritionist or trainer to help you get there.

4. **Stay connected to one another.** E-mail your group when a box of chocolates starts calling your name, or call them to say, "Hey, let's all go for a walk today."

5. **Celebrate successes!** Cheer group members on when they say no to a slice of birthday cake, run farther than they ever have on the treadmill, or shed even half a pound.

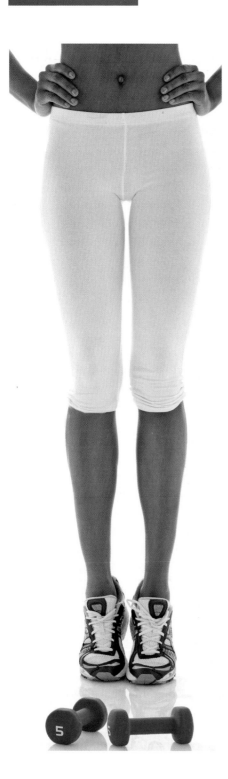

Surefire Solutions to Your Diet + Exercise Dilemmas

Too busy. No money. Don't want to mess up your hair. These are just a few of the excuses we use to avoid making fitness and healthy eating a part of our routine. We asked the experts to address your most common concerns. The next time you hear a voice in your head saying "I can't because..." try some of their inspiring comebacks. »

You say: "I'm too busy to go to the gym."

They say: Go old school, or take your workout with you. You don't need the latest gym machines to keep in shape, says celebrity trainer Kacy Duke. Phys-Ed conditioning—sit-ups, push-ups, lunges and squats, the stuff you learned in grade school—will get you good results. If you're on the road, says Duke, author of *The Show It Love Workout* (McGraw-Hill), "pack a jump rope or resistance bands in your suitcase."

You say: "Eating right is too expensive and time-consuming."

They say: Use your club card. "The best way to save money is to buy in bulk," says Aisha Cowart, director of personal training, nutrition and group conditioning for the Eastern Athletic clubs in New York. Cowart suggests taking advantage of discounters like BJ's, Sam's Club and Costco. Pick up cases of bottled water, lemons and limes to enhance that water, 100-calorie snack packs, and flavor boosters like olives and tomatoes. To save time, skip the prep steps by buying prewashed greens, cutup veggies and fresh fruit salads. Pack healthy snacks the night before, Cowart says, so in the morning, you can just grab and go.

You say: "All that sweating will wreck my hair!"

They say: Not all exercises will have your heart racing (think flexing yoga and toning Pilates), but when you do break a sweat, make sure to remove the perspiration from your hair, says Mikki Taylor, ESSENCE's beauty director and cover editor. "The salt residue can leave strands dry and brittle," she says. "You don't have to shampoo every time you work out, but you should at least rinse." Add a leave-in conditioner to coat and protect. Ultimately, you may need to change to a style that can accommodate frequent rinses and still look fly, Taylor says. Talk to your stylist about options like braids, locs, twists, a chignon or ponytail, or a short, workable cut.

You say: "I don't have any time to exercise."

They say: Sneak it in. Who says you have to get your 30 minutes in one block of time? Cowart gives this strategy to slip in your exercise throughout the day, whether you're home with the kids or on the job: Cardio can be 5 minutes of walking up and down the stairs plus 5 minutes of knee lifts in place. For toning, do 5 minutes of crunches plus 5 minutes of squats or lunges. Mix and match to sneak in three sets throughout your day.

You say: "Working out gets so tedious."

They say: Mix it up. "If you do the same thing all the time, your body will grow accustomed to it, and you'll get bored," Duke says. She offers these ways to jump-start a tired routine:

* Break up your normal run on the treadmill with half biking and half weight training.

* Step up your regular walk by running for 10 seconds then walking for 20. Gradually extend the run time until you're consistently challenging your heart to work harder.

* Ditch your circuit for a day and try something different like yoga or dance.

* Get a trainer who can show you new moves and help you target trouble spots.

* Take a break for a day or two. "Sometimes the best thing you can do is let the body rest," Duke says.

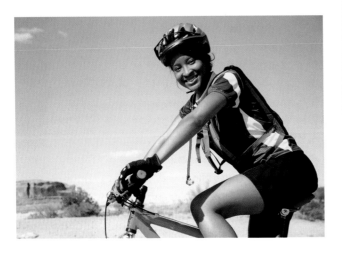

You say: "I'm too heavy (and embarrassed) to exercise."

They say: Go where you're comfortable. That could mean beginning with 10 minutes of dancing to your own iPod playlist in the comfort of your home or finding a female-friendly gym where people look like you, says Dallas R. Fuentes, owner of Perfect Parts Pilates, Inc., in New York.

You say: "I'm always hungry."

They say: Know which hunger you're feeding. "Your stomach is the size of a fist, so it doesn't take that much to fill it and feel full," Fuentes says. "When you're sincerely hungry, you hear and feel the acids in your stomach churning." When that's not happening but you want to eat, she says, "You need to ask yourself, 'What's not satisfied?'"

You say: "I want to be curvy, not cut."

They say: Think tight, not might. Experts say it's difficult for women to bulk up, even if we lift heavy weights, because we lack testosterone in the amounts that give men mass. "Don't fall for the old wives tale that exercise will make you muscle-bound," Cowart says. If you're still concerned, "do more repetitions with less weight," she suggests.

You say: "I would rather sleep than get up and be active."

They say: Imagine the feeling of getting it done. "It's the end goal that really motivates us," says Julia Griggs Havey, coauthor of *The Vice-Busting Diet* (St. Martin's Press). "The minute you push past the discomfort, it will be the best workout you ever had." Staying under the covers may make you feel better for half an hour, but an invigorating workout will make you feel better all day.

You say: "I do well for a while, then I get off track."

They say: Get back on as soon as you can. It's okay to have a bad day, or even a bad week or two, Duke says. It's even alright to eat something that's not so good for you every once in awhile. But a slip-up is not an invitation to give up. Add a fourth day of walking to your three-day schedule, or reduce your calorie intake for a few days, Duke suggests, and talk yourself back in the right direction. If you slipped because you stopped seeing results, you may have hit a plateau and need to adjust your goals accordingly, says New Jersey–based trainer and fitness consultant Benita Perkins. "You're probably no longer working hard enough," she says. Another word for that: progress.

You say: "I can't help but blow my diet when I eat out."

They say: Plan ahead. "These days most restaurants have menus online," says Kendell Hogan, West Coast regional fitness director at CRUNCH and host of ExerciseTV and ESPN's *Bodyshaping*. Some menus even give nutritional info, making it easier to choose wisely. "Check out the menu before you go, and you'll know ahead of time what you want," he says. Another option: Eat something at home in advance, then order light when dining out and skip dessert.

You say: "There's no park or safe area to be active."

They say: Take it inside, then take it to the streets. This is a serious issue for so many of us who live in urban areas. For the short-term, get yourself some DVDs and exercise indoors, and try to organize a program at your church. Perkins suggests encouraging a member of the church's praise dance group to take the lead. "It's worth the $300 to $500 investment to get that person certified to teach," she says. A longer-term strategy? Become an activist. Contact local community agencies and lawmakers to help improve your parks and designate safer, clean areas for outdoor activities, and get neighbors to join your cause.

"I Walked It Off!"

She put one foot in front of the other—and lost 92 pounds.

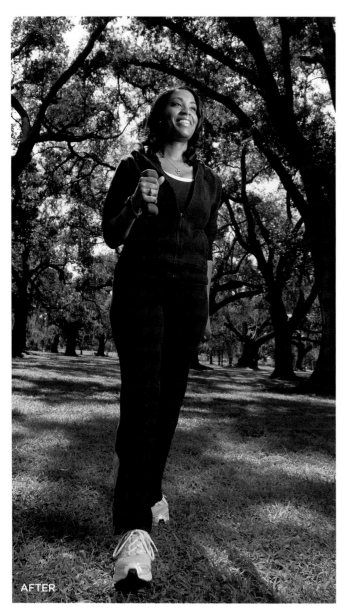

AFTER

MALEKA BEAL, 33
HEIGHT: 5' 3"
BEFORE: 230 lbs
AFTER: 138 lbs

Hurricane Katrina affected Maleka Beal of Louisiana in a surprising way. She and her husband, Eric, had to relocate to Texas for a while, all while caring for two sons and keeping a graphic design business up and running. She soon found that the storm had also uprooted her feelings about her health. Beal had always been full-figured. The faddish exercise equipment she bought, and eventually gave away, and all the diets she tried hadn't worked. Just before Katrina, she had given up trying to slim down. She decided she was happy with her body. After Katrina, she took a different view. "Suffering that type of loss really changes you," says Beal, who began to rethink the po'boys and fried chicken she freely ate. "It boiled down to being here as long as the love allowed and being here for our kids."

Beal and her husband started walking together two-and-a half miles a day, a welcome time for them to reconnect after living through such a tragedy. Once the walking got easier, they added hand and ankle weights, and then did a walk–run combination to switch up their workout routine. In about a year, Beal has lost more than 90 pounds and dropped from a size 18 to a size 4. Now back in New Orleans, Beal says, "When we reintroduce ourselves to friends or business associates, everybody is floored."

Sometimes, when Beal is extra busy and can't go for a walk, she'll just get down on the floor in her office and do some push-ups in her skirt and heels. "It's not that you have to work out for an hour straight," Beal says. "It's that ten or 15 minutes you give yourself, wherever you are." She has also committed herself to consuming just 1,500 calories a day. She gave up her favorite snack—vanilla ice cream on top of an apple pie straight out of the oven, with a little whipped cream. Now she eats Kashi cereals for breakfast instead of Burger King egg-and-cheese croissants. And she whips up dinners for her family with brown rice or whole wheat pasta, vegetables or salad and lean meat such as fish or chicken. "I'm changing my lifestyle and I'm changing my thought processes," says Beal, who admits the hardest part is getting up early to exercise. "I'm not saying it's easy, but I do it." As a result, Beal says that she's reaped an unexpected benefit: "My sex life is the best it has ever been!"

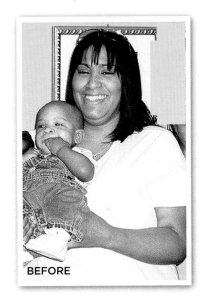

BEFORE

Expert's Advice: Mix Routines to Stay Committed

Beal found her motivation and kept it up, but success like hers can be short-lived if you don't constantly vary your workout, says Debbie Rocker, author of *Training for Life: Walk Your Way to Fitness and Weight Loss in 14 Days* (Springboard Press). She recommends taking off one day a week and mixing up your walk routine on all other days.

WAYS TO VARY YOUR WORKOUT:

Day 1:	Do 15-to-20-minute speed intervals as part of your walking routine.
Day 2:	Add lunges, sit-ups, squats or push-ups to your walk.
Day 3:	Take a 60-minute trek and add some hills.

The ESSENCE Total Body Fitness Challenge

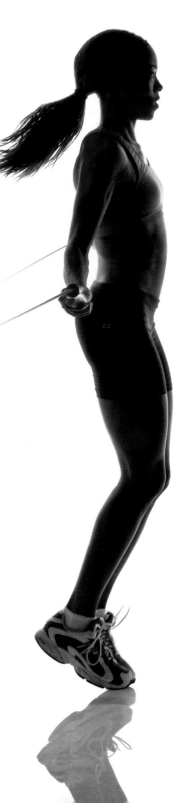

Give us 20 to 30 minutes and we'll give you a healthier heart, stronger arms, a toned tummy, firmer thighs and a butt so fabulous that gravity won't stand a chance! Start with our 20-minute cardio-strength Total Body Workout a few times a week, then on another day or two, add some moves from the following routines to target spots that need extra attention. Within a few weeks' time, you'll see results you'll love. »

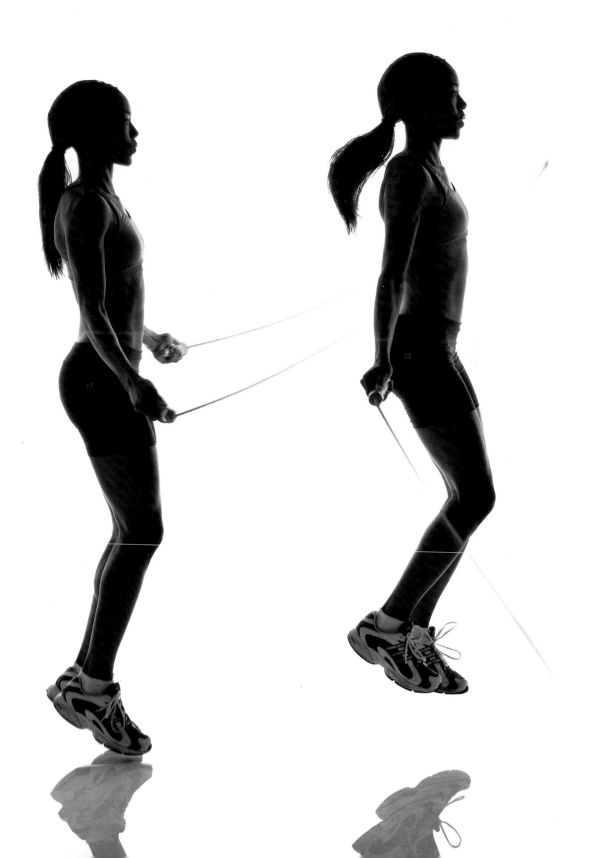

20 Minute Total Body Workout: Quick + Simple

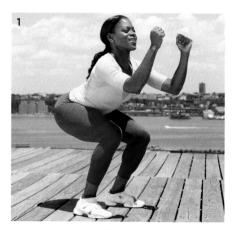

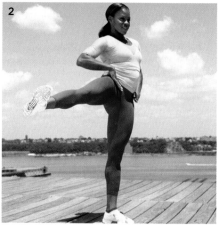

For your heart-pumping, muscle-strengthening foundation, we asked Bally Total Fitness expert Nikki Kimbrough to develop and demonstrate a quick, effective total-body workout that doesn't require equipment. Do this workout three times a week to boost your energy level and stay in shape. ≫

Squat Side Lift

WORKS BUTT, HIPS, INNER + OUTER THIGHS

STEP 1: Stand with feet hip width apart, and descend into a squat. Keep knees behind toes and abs tight. Extend arms forward with elbows slightly bent.

STEP 2: Raise upper body and place hands on hips while kicking right leg to the side with foot flexed. Kick as high as you can without losing balance. Return right foot to floor and resume squat position. Do two sets of ten on right leg, then switch to the left leg.

Power March

TONES THIGHS, CALVES, BUTT + ARMS

Stand with back erect, arms at sides, and hands in loose fists. As you breathe deeply, march quickly, pumping arms in an exaggerated motion for a slow count of 50. (If space is tight, march in place.) Pause and then repeat.

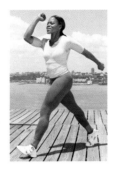

✻ FIT TIP: Exercise reduces symptoms of anxiety and depression, according to the Centers for Disease Control. Researchers aren't sure why but suspect that it's the rush of feel-good endorphins and the drop in stress-mongering cortisol.

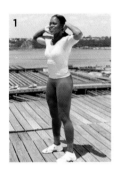
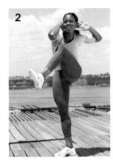

Knee Lifts

SCULPTS HIPS + ABS

STEP 1: Stand with feet hip width apart and knees soft. Clasp hands loosely behind your head so that elbows are facing outward.

STEP 2: Twist torso to the left, and with foot flexed, raise left knee toward chest. Point right elbow toward left knee. Return to starting position. Repeat exercise, this time with left elbow pointing toward right knee. Do two to three sets of 15

Lateral Jumps

STRENGTHENS THIGHS + ARMS

STEP 1: Stand erect with feet together, elbows bent, shoulders relaxed and hands balled into fists at sides. (Kick this move up a notch by holding a three-to-five-pound weight in each hand.) With legs and feet together and arms in starting position, hop about ten inches to the right. Land with knees slightly bent.

STEP 2: Now jump ten inches to the left. Do two sets of 15.

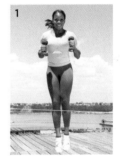
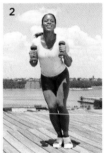

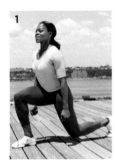
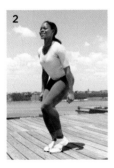

Lunge Step-ups

TARGETS THIGHS, ABS + GLUTES

STEP 1: Start in a lunge position keeping back erect.

STEP 2: As you slowly raise upper body, pull left leg forward to meet right. Continue to keep knees slightly bent and back straight. Return to starting position and repeat on same side. Do two sets of 12 reps on both sides. (If you feel off balance, lightly rest a hand on the back of a sofa or along a wall.)

Pilates: Tone + Strengthen

With its muscle-firming movements and deep, calming breaths, Pilates burns fat even after you put away the mat, says Jeanette Jenkins, a Pilates instructor and president of The Hollywood Trainer in Los Angeles. "Your body uses fat as fuel to recharge the muscles you've worked," she explains. She shows the Pilates routine she created exclusively for ESSENCE. >>

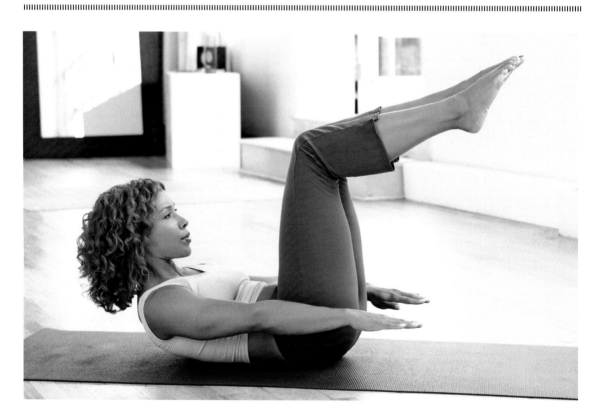

The Hundred

FLATTENS YOUR BELLY

Lie down, raising your head and shoulders off the ground. With legs together, bend and lift knees so calves are parallel to the floor. Then, quickly pump arms downward five times. With each pump, draw in a quick breath. Now for another count of five, pump arms and push air out. Do nine more sets for a total of a hundred pumps.

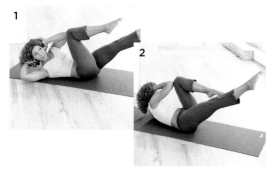

Obliques

GOOD FOR SIDES OF TORSO

STEP 1: Lie on your back, place hands behind your head, and raise shoulders off the floor. Bend knees to lift calves parallel to the floor. Inhale, twist torso to the right, bring left elbow and right knee together, and straighten left leg. STEP 2: Switch sides and repeat. For next rep, exhale. Continue for two sets of 12.

Double Leg Stretch

TIGHTENS ABS

STEP 1: Lie on your back, with arms at sides and head resting on floor. Lift head and shoulders up, pull knees into chest, and reach forward so fingertips touch ankles. STEP 2: Exhale and touch shoulders; straighten arms as you straighten legs. As you inhale, sweep arms in a circular motion and return them to starting position. Do six reps.

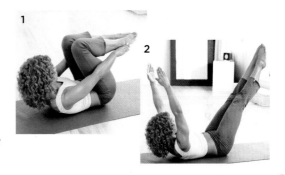

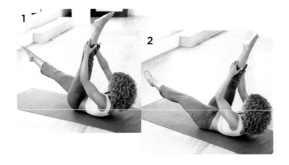

Scissors

WORKS THIGH MUSCLES + STRENGTHENS ABS

STEP 1: Lie on your back, with shoulders and head off the floor. Lift right leg; grasp left leg with both hands. As you exhale, pull left leg toward chest for two pulses. STEP 2: Inhale and switch sides, grasping right leg and straightening left leg. Exhale while reaching for the right leg for two pulses. Do two sets of eight.

Leg Lift

SCULPTS SHOULDERS, ARMS, THIGHS + LOWER ABS

STEP 1: With palms and heels planted on floor, legs together and toes pointed, raise hips and butt. STEP 2: Inhale and lift right leg 12 inches off the floor. Exhale, and as you flex right foot, return right leg to starting position. To complete rep, repeat move with left leg. Do two sets of eight reps.

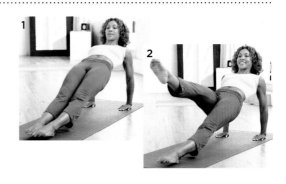

Armed+ Fabulous

Bally expert Nikki Kimbrough gives you a workout to firm up your biceps and triceps and tone that upper body. »

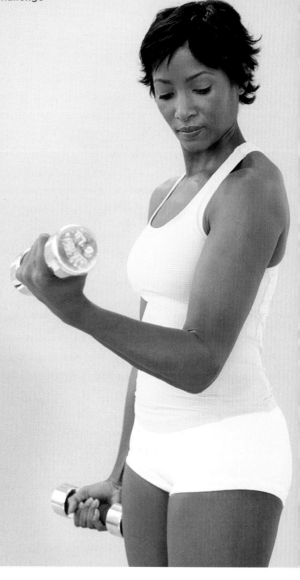

Biceps Curls

STRENGTHENS BICEPS

Stand with feet shoulder width apart and back erect. Grasp a three- or five-pound dumbbell in each hand; place arms at sides and palms facing upward. Now slowly curl right arm up toward shoulder and back down. Repeat on left. Do three sets of 10 to 12 reps.

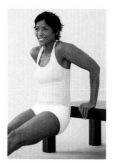

Seated Dips

TONES TRICEPS + UPPER BACK

Sit in a hard stationary chair or bench with arms behind you and hands gripping the edge of the seat. Walk legs out in front of you until your butt is suspended directly in front of the seat, then plant heels on the floor and flex feet. Now, keeping your elbows at your sides and your core muscles tight, slowly lower butt as close to the floor as possible. Pause, then slowly push yourself up until your arms are straight. Do two sets of six to eight reps until you build the strength to complete two sets of ten to 12 reps.

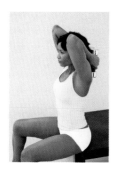

Overhead Triceps Extension
TONES TRICEPS + UPPER BACK

Holding a three- or five-pound dumbbell in each hand, sit at the edge of stationary chair or bench with your back erect and legs shoulder width apart.Extend arms over your head so that the weights and your palms are facing each other. To complete rep, slowly lower dumbbells behind your head, bending elbows until they are pointing toward the ceiling and your biceps are nearly touching your forearms. Return to starting position and repeat. Do three sets of 10 to 12 reps.

Lateral Pulls
WORKS ARMS, SHOULDERS + BACK

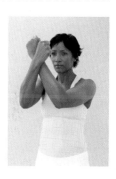

Stand keeping back straight, chest lifted, abdominal muscles contracted and shoulders relaxed. Ball your hands into fists, then cross right wrist over left. Then, while keeping your wrists crossed, slowly raise your arms over your head, contracting the upper-back muscles. Hold for a few seconds. Then as you press your shoulder blades together, slowly lower elbows until your fists are in front of shoulders. Return arms overhead, cross wrists, and repeat. Do two sets of 10 to 12 reps.

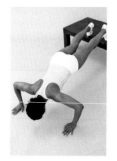

Elevated Push-Ups
STRENGTHENS CHEST, SHOULDERS + TRICEPS

Get into push-up position with head in line with spine. Place the balls of your feet on the seat of a stationary chair or bench. (If you are at the gym, use a two- or three-rise step bench.) Bend elbows and lower upper body until your nose hovers over the floor. Keep your core muscles tight to avoid injury and to benefit fully from the move. Then slowly straighten elbows and return to starting position. Start with two sets of six to eight reps. Work up to three sets of 10 to 12.

Wrist Curls
STRENGTHENS WRISTS + FOREARMS

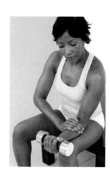

Sit on the edge of stationary chair or bench with feet flat on the floor and legs parted. Grasp a three- or five-pound dumbbell with your left hand. Lean forward, resting right forearm on upper thigh so that left hand is extended just beyond the knee. Place right hand on top of left forearm to hold it in place. Now curl right wrist upward without moving either forearm. Complete rep by lowering weight until your right wrist is fully flexed. Do two sets of ten to 12 reps. Repeat on the right side.

Bring Up the Rear

Bottom need a lift? Don't worry. "Strengthening the lower body can raise the rear so it appears more shapely," says Bally Fitness expert Nikki Kimbrough. Work these no-fail moves to tone and lift your tush. »

The Twist

SHAPES TORSO, REAR + LEGS

Place arms at shoulder level, with right forearm in front of chest. In a semisquat, with feet pointed right, jut hip out to left side. Then jump, crossing arms in front of chest. Land, with right hip out, feet pointed left, and left forearm in front of chest. Jump to return to starting position for one rep. Do two sets of 12 reps.

The Sexy Squeeze

TONES REAR + LOWER BACK

STEP 1: With feet shoulder width apart, toes forward and hands on hips, glance at your bottom as you arch your back and then jut your rear out behind you.

STEP 2: Squeezing butt, contract abs to push pelvis forward for one rep. Do two sets of ten to 12 reps.

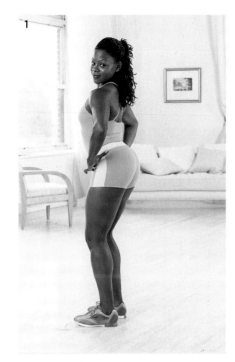

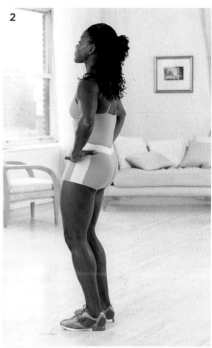

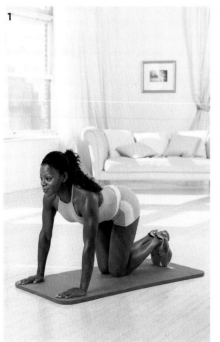

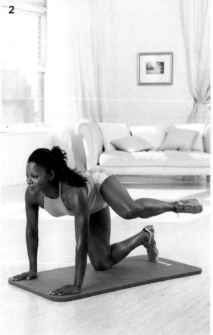

Fire-Me-Ups

WORKS LOWER BACK, HIPS, BUTT + LEGS

STEP 1: Kneel down on all fours. Keep back straight and head looking forward.

STEP 2: Raise left knee to shoulder level, lower and repeat. On tenth rep, keep knee in air and pump it up slightly higher ten times. Then lower. Repeat on right side for one set. Do a total of two sets.

Gentle Moves

Strong, flexible muscles, which keep joints aligned, are the building blocks of good posture and pain-free movement. Here, Renée Daniels, certified medical exercise specialist and coauthor of *Straighter, Stronger, Leaner, Longer* (Avery), shows you how to get them. »

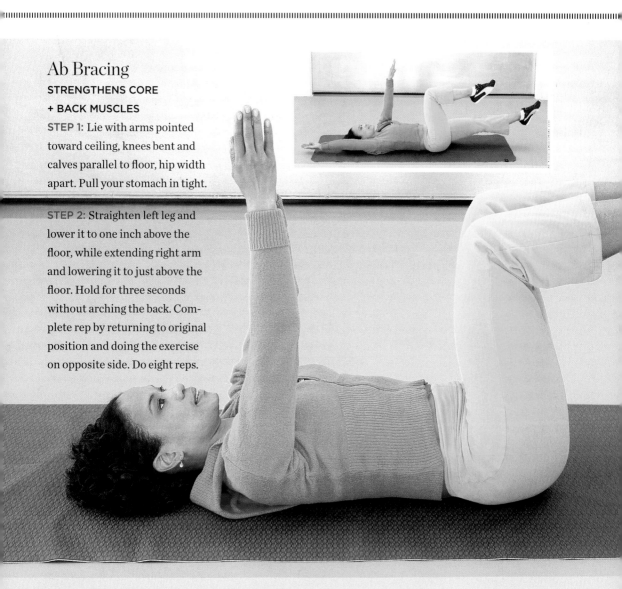

Ab Bracing

STRENGTHENS CORE + BACK MUSCLES

STEP 1: Lie with arms pointed toward ceiling, knees bent and calves parallel to floor, hip width apart. Pull your stomach in tight.

STEP 2: Straighten left leg and lower it to one inch above the floor, while extending right arm and lowering it to just above the floor. Hold for three seconds without arching the back. Complete rep by returning to original position and doing the exercise on opposite side. Do eight reps.

Angel Squeeze

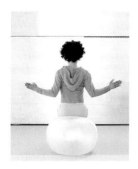

REAR SHOULDER MUSCLES

Sit with your back straight on an exercise ball or in a chair, place your legs hip width apart and leave your feet flat on the floor. Bend elbows and hold them at chest level. Press forearms and palms together. Next open arms to each side as you squeeze shoulder blades together as if you're crushing a can between them. Finally, with back straight, lower elbows to waist while lifting chest up to ceiling. Return to original position. Do ten to 12 reps.

Side Bend

LOWER BACK + HIP MUSCLES

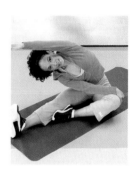

While sitting on the floor, extend right leg with a flexed foot, but bend left knee and bring your left foot to touch your right knee. Cross your right hand over to touch your left knee and straighten left arm out to the side with fingertips touching floor. Lift left arm over head and reach diagonally toward the right foot. As you lift, turn head to the left and look toward ceiling, but don't strain. Hold this position for three seconds and then return back to start. Do five reps, then repeat on other side.

Rope Stretch

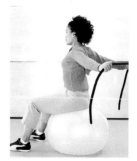

LOOSENS CHEST + IMPROVES POSTURE

Sit on exercise ball or chair with your legs hip width apart, your feet flat on the floor, and your back straight. Grasp the ends of a rope or towel with both hands. Without shrugging your shoulders, lift arms straight up over head keeping them a little wider than shoulder width apart. While maintaining straight arms, extend reach behind you. Hold stance for three or four seconds, then return arms to previous overhead position. Do five reps.

The Clam

STRENGTHENS HIPS

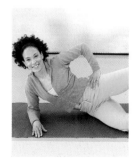

Lie on the floor on your right side, with knees stacked and bent and your left hand propped on your hip. Use your right elbow to support your upper body. Lift left leg, rotating knee toward ceiling. Use the hand on your hip to make sure you avoid rolling your hips back as you rotate the top leg. Hold for three or four seconds while squeezing hip and butt muscles. Lower leg to starting position. Do one set of 10 reps on each side. Work up to three sets.

Top Fitness Strategies for Every Age

No matter how many candles are on your birthday cake, experts recommend vigorous exercise 30 minutes a day at least six days a week—and admit even three days of 20 minutes is worthwhile. But a fitness plan that works for you at 22 won't be right when you're 47. Here are workouts that our experts recommend, decade by decade. Consult your doctor before you begin a new regime, and include gentle warm-up and cool-down stretches. >>

AGE

>> Your 20s

"You can do more dynamic and aerobic work now," says Aisha Cowart, director of personal training, nutrition and group counseling at Eastern Athletic clubs in New York. Try to develop habits to last the rest of your life.

>> Your 30s

Your energy may be sapped by motherhood, relationships and work. So do double duty: Put the baby in a stroller and go for a walk, or try a belly dancing class with your girlfriends.

>> Your 40s

Hormonal shifts cause your metabolism to slow, bone density to decline and your waist to expand. Resistance workouts counter muscle and bone-density loss, Pilates can target your waist, and water exercises are easy on joints.

>> Your 50s + Beyond

After menopause comes loss of bone density, which does a number on your posture. If you've never picked up a weight, it's not too late: Strengthen your bones and protect yourself from falls and fractures.

AEROBIC	STRENGTH	FLEXIBILITY
Capoeira Spinning Kickboxing Running Jump-rope circuit Zumba In-line skating	Basic Training Boot camp Circuit work	Ashtanga or Bikram yoga Pilates mat Budokon
Running Cardio boxing Hip-hop dance Latin dancing Belly dancing Skating Biking	Resist-a-ball Integrated movement Free weights	Pilates mat Vinyassa yoga
Jogging African dance Latin dancing Modern/jazz dance Biking Step aerobics Water aerobics	NIA (blend of tai chi, yoga, dance and martial arts) Cardio sculpt Agility circuit	Kundalini or Iynegar yoga Gyrotronics Pilates Reformer
Power walking Belly dancing Broadway dance Stationary biking Aquatics	Free weights Basic circuit work Body Bar work Resistance bands or tubes	Hatha or restorative yoga Tai chi Pilates mat

Cross-train for Maximum Results

No matter what your age, the components of keeping fit are:

Strength: your ability to bear weight and apply force (pushing, pulling)

Endurance: the extent to which you can sustain intense aerobic activity (running, cycling)

Flexibility: the range of motion of your joints (bending, stretching)

Keep this balance in mind as you mix different exercises. Alternating strength, aerobic and flexibility workouts—also known as cross-training—not only improves your overall fitness, but also helps you reduce the risk of injury because you avoid stressing the same muscles and joints each day. Plus, the variety should keep you challenged.

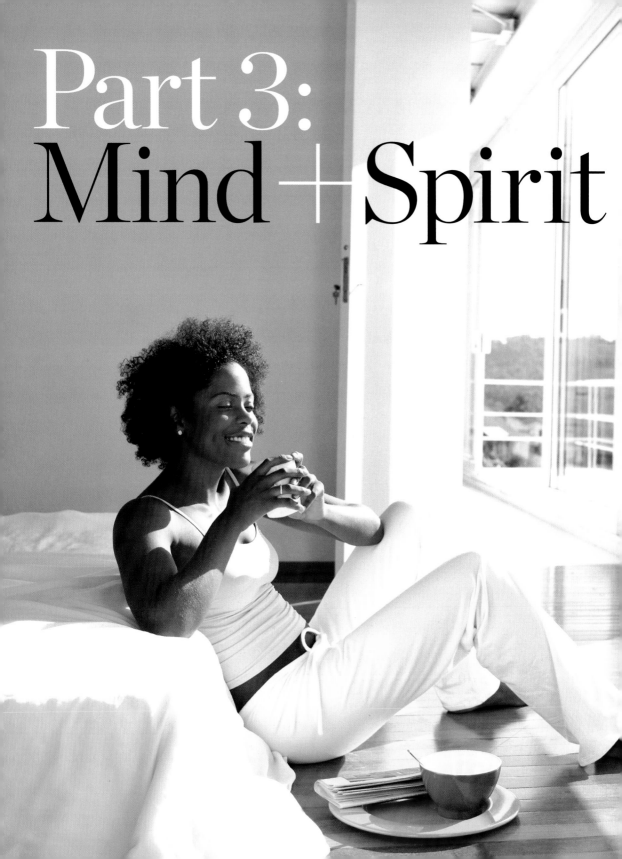

Part 3:
Mind+Spirit

No More Stress

Ever walked into a room and forgot what you were there for? Or had to wear your swimsuit under your work suit because you ran out of time to do laundry? Ever snapped at your little one for wanting some attention when yours was already spent? Or popped Tylenol like they were Mike and Ikes to fix that nagging headache? Yes, you have that project due at work, and the church hospitality committee meeting to lead, and you still have to check in on your grand-aunt, get dinner on the table and see your child through another night of homework. Black women are prone to piling it on, but doing too much can stress you out. Studies have shown that chronic stress not only causes headaches, body pain and depression, but can contribute to immune disorders, diabetes, cancer and heart disease. This section will show you how to push away from the Table of Too Much; explore holistic, natural and spiritual options for conquering stress; and give you the best advice from Black doctors on what to do when the blues just won't let you go. Oh, and remember that time you went to work with the curler still in the back of your head? Repeat after us: Never again. »

Just Say *Aahhh!*

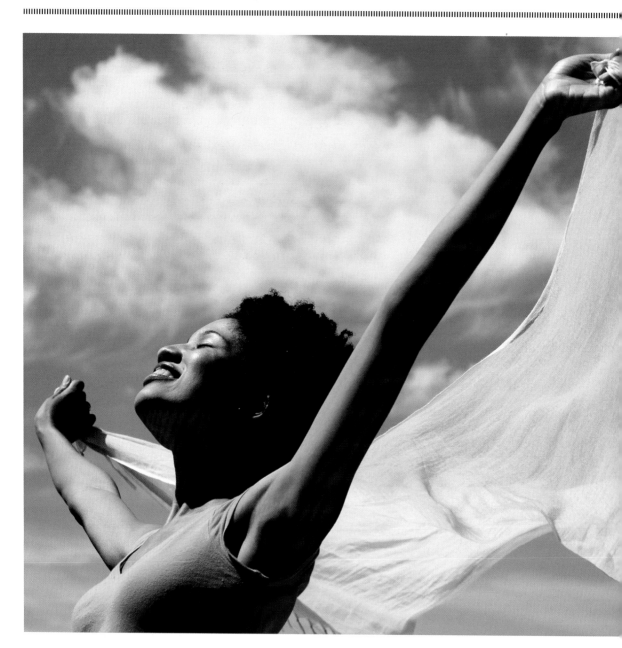

Too many of us feel neither able nor entitled to do anything about how chronically overextended we are. Give yourself permission to slow down. Here are some paths to inner peace that you may not have considered. »

Unpaid bills. Single parenting. Working two jobs. Taking care of too many folks and too many problems. People might call us "Superwomen," but carrying the weight of the world is a heavy burden. Consider what crushng stress is doing to your body: Adrenaline floods your system; your blood pressure skyrockets; and your heart rate accelerates, taxing your arteries. Your liver pumps excess glucose into your bloodstream, raising your risk for diabetes, and fat cells rush to conserve energy, making it easier to gain weight. Over time, plaque accumulates in your blood vessels, setting you up for heart disease and strokes. Constant anxiety also inundates your system with glucocorticoids (including the stress hormone, cortisol), which suppress immunity, impair memory and cognitive function, and signal your body to deposit energy-storing fat cells around your middle, further challenging your heart. It's why we're more likely than other groups to suffer from heart disease, stroke, obesity, cancer and diabetes. And it's why so many of us live with our emotions perpetually set on a hair trigger. But it doesn't have to be this way. Practices like acupuncture, meditation, massage, aromatherapy, yoga and reflexology can reduce stress and promote relaxation with lasting benefits. If we can't eliminate all our stressors, we can at least master our responses to them. Just remember, these techniques are not a substitute for traditional care, so let your doctor know you're practicing alternative therapies.

"Carve out a period today to do absolutely nothing. It might be 20 minutes or an hour. Sit or lie somewhere comfortable and pleasant, and just be." —LIFE COACH VALORIE BURTON

Scent Sense: Aromatherapy

We know that certain smells—fresh- baked cookies, wet grass, the scent of a newborn baby—can bring a flood of positive emotions. That's the theory behind aromatherapy, which uses highly concentrated scented oils, derived from distilling or cold-pressing plants and flowers, to affect disposition. "You can have a change in mood within a few seconds," says Raphael d'Angelo, M.D., president of the International Alliance of Aromatherapists. D'Angelo who incorporates aromatherapy into his medical practice, has found aromatherapy useful in treating everything from respiratory illnesses to infection.

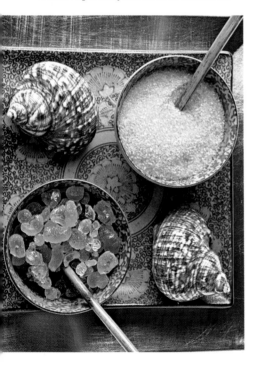

How It Works

The aromatherapist will ask about your lifestyle and any medical issues, then will mix various oils to address your concerns. For instance, if you complain of stress, she might mix oil of geranium, said to have balancing properties, with lavender to calm and soothe. The essential oils may then be blended with another unscented oil, such as almond, and used in a massage so that the benefits are absorbed into the skin. Or the blend may be put in a diffuser to scent the room. Some studies have shown lavender, lemon and vanilla to be effective in elevating mood and helping with insomnia and even anxiety. Other popular aromatherapy oils are peppermint, said to be useful in treating headaches; eucalyptus, used for treating respiratory problems such as colds or asthma; and ylang-ylang, which is supposed to ease anxiety.

Try This at Home

Put a few drops of lavender in your bath for a relaxing soak before bed. Or scent your home with essential oils placed in a diffuser or nebulizer. You can also combine drops of essential oil with some water in a spray bottle and mist the air around you.

Resources

While there are no licensing requirements for aromatherapists in the United States, the Alliance of International Aromatherapists will supply you with contact information for a trained therapist in your area: alliance-aroma therapists.org; 303-531-6377. Keep in mind that conclusive studies have yet to be done on the effectiveness of some oils that are currently in use. For more on essential oils that may alleviate your specific ailments, visit aromaweb.com.

A Quiet Mind: Meditation

Meditation is one of the simplest, most inexpensive and effective methods of stress reduction. Studies show regular meditation can lower blood pressure, ease depression and anxiety, and help deal with chronic pain. All you need is a quiet place and some time—anywhere from 5 to 45 minutes—to clear the clutter from your mind. There are several methods of meditation, all of them based on the principle that if you gently steer your mind away from thoughts of the past and future—the chores still to be done, tomorrow's meeting with your boss, the fight you had with your partner—you can achieve serenity. It's not only happiness that improves with meditation, which has its roots in Eastern spirituality. Many people claim that a regular meditation practice also helps them deal with life's random frustrations. "You become mindful of what you're thinking," says Joseph Schmidt, executive director of New York Insight Meditation Center. "Mindfulness puts a break on the negative cycles of stress that people fall into."

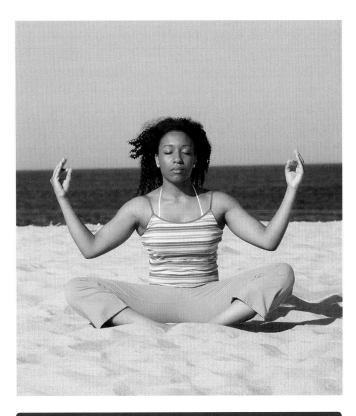

Resources **Most major cities have meditation centers. For a variety of meditations you can try, visit meditationcenter.com.**

How It Works

The key to meditation is consistency. You can practice on your own or use a meditation CD. Beginners may benefit from a guided sitting at a meditation center. Students rest on a cushion, bench or chair while the teacher encourages each participant to focus on the sound of her or his breathing or an image or other sound.

Try This at Home

Pick a time, place and duration—a rule of thumb is five minutes more than is comfortable. Starting with your scalp, mentally release tension from each part of your body. Focus on your breath or repeat a phrase in your mind, such as "I am peaceful." When another thought or emotion enters your mind, gently push it away.

Foot Notes: Reflexology

There is nothing more soothing at the end of a long day than having someone rub your aching feet. And as talented as your man may be at this intimate gesture, every woman deserves to have her feet worked by a pro. Reflexology is based on the idea that various parts of our feet correspond with different parts of our body—for instance, the tips of the toes reflect the head, and the balls of the feet reflect the heart. By applying pressure to points on the foot, reflexologists aim to affect the corresponding body part. While some may question the science, the practice has been used to treat everything from menstrual cramps and labor pains to anxiety and depression. "Reflexology is so effective because within seconds of a treatment patients fall into a totally relaxed state," says Kevin Kunz, author, along with his wife, Barbara, of 11 books on reflexology. Many people think of reflexology as an Asian practice, but evidence of footwork can be found in all major cultures from Native American to African, says Kunz, who is based in Albuquerque, New Mexico. In the 1900's, a Connecticut doctor charted the nerve pathways of the body. Later, physical therapist Eunice Ingham took up his research, mapping out areas of the foot and creating the diagrams used by reflexologists today.

How It Works

At your first appointment, you will be asked to give a medical history and to share any physical ailments or concerns. You will then remove your shoes and socks and lie on a massage table or in a comfortable chair. The therapist will cradle your foot with one hand and use the other to apply pressure. A session may last from 30 minutes to an hour. While you might feel a slight tenderness in certain areas, you should never feel pain. "The treatment should never go beyond your comfort zone," Kunz says.

Try This at Home

Try putting some small rubber balls in an old sock and rolling your feet over the balls. Or purchase a foot roller and keep it under your desk for a midday treat.

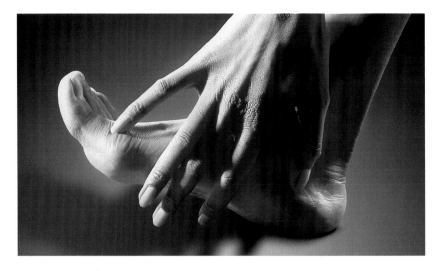

Resources

To find a qualified reflexologist in your area, visit the International Institute of Reflexology's referral list at reflexology-usa.net; 727-343-4811.

Good Point: Acupuncture

Acupuncture is based on the belief that energy, or Qi (pronounced "chee"), flows through our body along pathways, or meridians, that can sometimes get blocked. "It's like electricity," says Gena Spencer, a Sacramento, California–based licensed acupuncturist who has been practicing for 11 years. "We can't see it, but we know it's there. If you have a smooth flow of Qi, then your circulation, immune system and nervous system will work better." The meridians can be accessed and opened up through different points along the pathway. The acupuncture practitioner stimulates these points with fine metallic needles, which are disposed of after use. Traditional Eastern and Western practitioners use acupuncture to treat a range of conditions from menopause to asthma. Research has shown acupuncture to be successful in treating pain, depression, drug addiction and infertility. Spencer regularly treats African-American women who complain of anxiety. "Stress manifests in many different ways, from not sleeping and panic attacks to headaches and overeating," she says. "Acupuncture can help with all of these things." Specific points are stimulated to influence the brain to release serotonin, one of the hormones that helps you deal with stress. Research suggests that acupuncture can also increase the body's production of endorphins, another feel-good hormone.

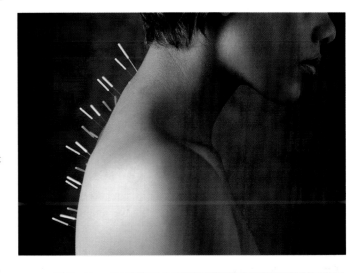

How It Works

A typical session lasts an hour. The acupuncturist takes your medical history, checks your pulse and looks at your tongue for signs of imbalance or illness. You then change into a gown and lie on a table. Sterile needles are inserted into your extremities, torso, neck or ears. The needles are almost as thin as a human hair and most people barely feel them. In fact, many people fall asleep.

Try This at Home

It is impossible to practice acupuncture on yourself. But you can try acupressure, which involves stimulating the acupoints with pressure instead of needles. For more information on how to administer acupressure, see Magic Touch: Massage (next page).

Resources For licensed acupuncturists in your area, check the American Association of Acupuncture and Oriental Medicine at aaaomonline.org; 866-455-7999.

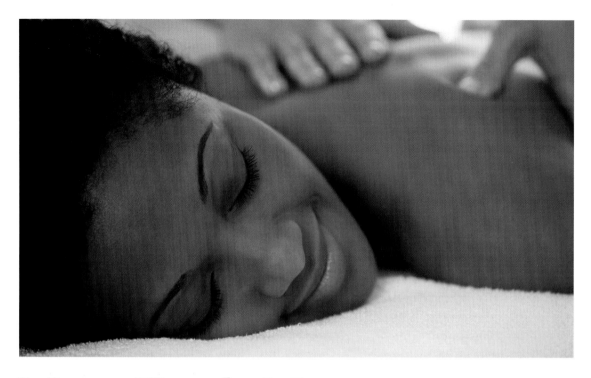

Magic Touch: Massage

You probably think of it as the most decadent indulgence, right up there with the rose-petal pedicure. But for the harried woman, a regular massage can work wonders. "When you're stressed, your body releases the hormone cortisol, which gets to your muscles and prompts them to create adhesions, which are like scar tissue," says Shannon Grant, a licensed massage therapist and owner of The Art of Touch Therapeutic Massage Center in Atlanta. "You can have adhesions in your shoulders and neck just from sitting at a desk all day. Adhesions can be very uncomfortable and affect your range of motion. Massage breaks up those adhesions and can bring a lot of relief." Studies also have shown that massage can reduce frequency of headaches; improve chronic back, neck and shoulder pain; ease premenstrual syndrome; aid in sleep; and even improve the function of your immune system. Grant says she's experienced the effects firsthand. "In massage school, as part of my training I would get massages three days a week," she remembers. "At the time, I felt great. I never got sick and had high energy. I didn't make the connection until I finished school, stopped getting massages and all the bad stuff came back." Now she's back to getting regular massages, and wants others to gain its benefits too.

Try This:

Can't afford an hour out of your day? Many nails salons offer ten-minute chair massages. Give yourself a treat.

How It Works

At your first appointment, the massage therapist will ask you for a brief medical history. It's especially important to mention any injuries, pain and bone or muscle problems. The therapist might ask you what kind of pressure you'd like, very deep or more of a gentle stroke. If you don't know, don't worry. The therapist will check in with you during the treatment to make sure you are comfortable. She will leave you alone in the treatment room to disrobe (you can leave on your panties if you like, but everything else should come off), and provide a blanket or sheet for you to cover yourself. She will work on one part of your body at a time, leaving the rest covered. If you'd prefer that she focus on a particular area, just let her know. A light oil or lotion will be used for the massage—be sure to mention any allergies—and the therapist may incorporate aromatherapy as well. If you prefer to see a male or female massage therapist, mention this when you make your appointment.

Try This at Home

You can massage your feet, hands, arms and legs yourself. But there's nothing like a good back rub—and for that you need another person. Trade massages with your partner. Lie on the floor and let him get to work. Another option: Get your child to help you out. There are plenty of handheld electronic back massagers that even a 6-year-old can operate.

Which Massage?

Here are some of the more popular massage techniques. Speak to your therapist about what might work best for you.

Swedish Perhaps the best-known Western technique, Swedish consists of kneading, stroking and stretching the layer of your muscles just below the skin's surface.
Good for: Relaxation and first-timers

Deep Tissue A massage therapist will work on a specific part of your body, such as your shoulders or lower back. The pressure is intense, and can be uncomfortable for someone wanting a lighter touch. **Good for:** Very tight muscles, chronic pain and injuries

Acupressure Think of it as acupuncture without the needles. Your body has hot spots called acupoints, which are located everywhere from your forehead to your palms to your feet. Eastern medicine holds that these acupoints can affect some organs and their functions. With this technique, pressure is applied to those acupoints through massage.
Good for: Relaxation, insomnia and menstrual cramps

Resources To find a qualified massage therapist in your area, check the American Massage Therapy Association at findamassagetherapist.org; 888-843-2682, or Associated Bodywork and Massage Professionals at massagetherapy.com; 800-458-2267. Or contact a local massage school and ask about programs where students, supervised by instructors, will treat you. They often do so at a reduced cost. When massage is used for pain management or as part of a physical therapy program, it may be partially covered by your insurance.

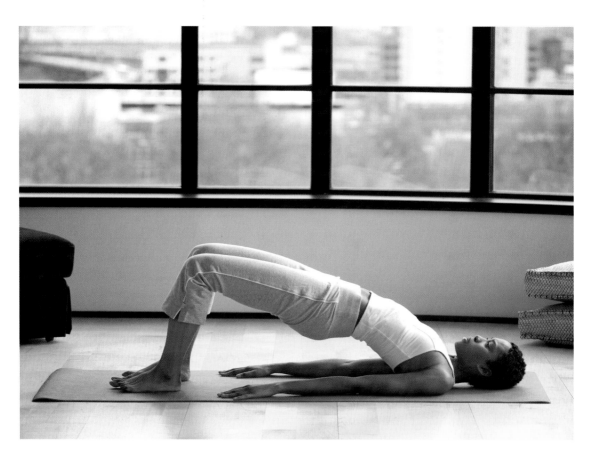

Deep Stretch: Yoga

Yoga comes from the Sanskrit word *yuj*, which means to unite, and the aim of yoga is to unite the mind, body and spirit. Physically, yoga increases flexibility and strength, and helps bring the body into proper alignment. For those of us who carry our stress in hunched-up shoulders and tight lower backs, yoga works wonders. But yoga also quiets the mind. Many classes are set to soothing new age music. And all classes pay special attention to the breath, with the instructor reminding you to inhale and exhale. "You'll never breathe as deeply as you do in a yoga class," says Ursula Scherrer, a certified yoga instructor in Manhattan. During a yoga class, a teacher may also ask you to concentrate on a particular part of your anatomy—spine, chest, inner thighs—as you sink into a pose. Christina Pearce, a yoga teacher in Brooklyn, says body awareness is particularly important for Black women. "Most of us weren't taught how to have a relationship with our bodies," she notes, "and yoga is such a good way to develop that."

How It Works

All yoga classes are composed of a series of poses, called asanas. Some classes move quickly and energetically from one pose to another while others move more slowly and fluidly. Some classes focus on holding a pose for a longer period of time; others are more concerned with the ways you can breathe during a pose. They all have in common the savasana (or corpse) pose, a five-to-ten-minute relaxation at the end of the class during which students lie faceup on their mats, eyes closed. The teacher may ask you to feel your body sinking into the ground as you focus on your breath. For many people the stillness of the pose is the most relaxing time of their day.

Wear nonrestrictive, comfortable clothing to class and bring a towel and some water. Your gym or yoga studio will provide a sticky mat to keep you from sliding, or you can bring your own (available at any sports store). If you have any aches or injuries, or are pregnant, let the instructor know before class begins.

Try This at Home

As with any exercise, the benefits of yoga come with consistency. If you can't make it to the gym as often as you'd like, try some of the excellent yoga DVDs or free podcasts, including a morning wake-up and an evening relaxation, on yogajournal.com.

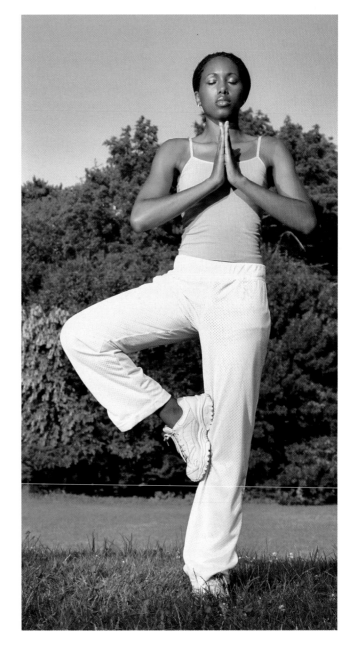

[Resources Yoga studios can be found in every major city, and most gyms now offer yoga classes.

Yoga Moves: Take Your Pick

There are many approaches to yoga. The key is finding a style that suits you. Most teachers will allow you to watch a class first. Notice if the teacher demonstrates the poses and circulates to offer instruction to class members. If she stays at the head of the room and calls out the poses, the class may be more advanced. Here's a quick guide to some of the more popular styles to help you find your match:

Hatha

The umbrella term for most yoga practiced in the West. If you see it on a class schedule, it usually refers to a slower-paced class that focuses on connecting the breath with the movements. **Good for:** Beginners

Ashtanga
(sometimes called "power yoga"):

A vigorous form of yoga in which the class moves energetically from one pose to another to build strength and endurance. There is little focus on meditation. **Good for:** An intense and challenging workout

Kundalini

The teacher guides the class through various breathing techniques in conjunction with specific poses. **Good for:** Vitality and increased energy

Vinyasa
(sometimes called "flow yoga"):

Focuses on moving fluidly from one pose to the next. The class will typically include a series of sun salutations and then move into more intense stretching. **Good for:** Relaxation and proper alignment

Iyengar

Focuses on proper alignment and holding poses for a longer period of time to achieve maximum benefits. **Good for:** Correcting posture and flexibility

Bikram
(also called "hot yoga"):

Practiced in a room heated up to 105 degrees. Each class moves through 26 poses in a specific order. Make sure to drink plenty of water the day before you go. **Good for:** Increasing flexibility and strength, and profuse sweating, which helps your body shed toxins

Restorative

A very gentle practice that makes use of props like belts, blocks and blankets to help students get into deeply relaxing poses to renew and heal the body. **Good for:** Relaxation or people with mobility issues

Hip Shake: African Dance

Sometimes the best way to blow off steam, calm your mind and free your spirit is to move. Twenty years ago, Darmone Holland, a wellness coach and dance and yoga instructor in Brooklyn, developed a popular African dance–based workout routine. "I wanted Black women to be able to get a cardio workout and experience movements that we could relate to," Holland says. "These are dances that were done by our ancestors. The movements are in our genes and resonate with us. For people of African descent, who can be so disconnected from their past, the sense of connection they find in an African dance class can be very healing."

African dance also offers Black women the opportunity to take a class where the instructor has a body type similar to their own. In African dance classes, they see a larger woman who looks like they do, moving with tremendous grace and power. "For African-American women, this can be very inspiring," Holland notes. "The woman teaching any class is setting the tone for what the class should be striving to look like." It doesn't hurt that all that movement is good for you. "When my class does African dance, they're moving and breaking a sweat and producing endorphins, which are also known as the happy hormones," Holland says.

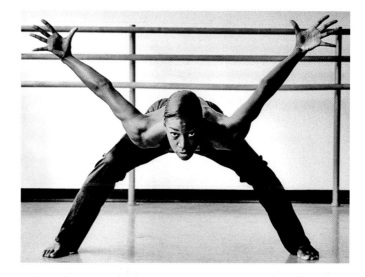

How It Works

Most African dance classes are taught in the West African tradition, accompanied by live drummers. Many of the dances are ceremonial and incorporate a lot of hip, back and arm movements. The class typically starts with warm-up stretches and simple moves, followed by vigorous choreography that makes for a great cardio workout, ending with a slower-paced stretch and cool down.

Try This at Home

You may not have done this since you were a teenager, but it's still just as much fun: Put on your favorite up-tempo music and dance! Do all the steps that you remember from back in the day—for as fast and for as long as you can.

Resources **Check your local gym, dance studio or creative arts center for African dance classes.**

We asked scholars, healers and spiritual leaders for their secrets to lasting joy. They helped us uncover these principles for emotional well-being. »

Your Pursuit of Happiness

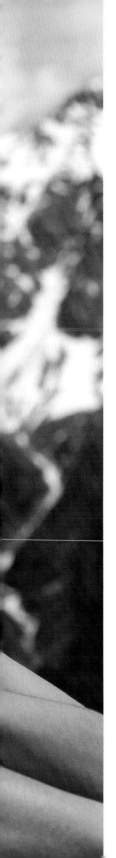

1} EMBRACE THE HERE AND NOW. Happiness need never be deferred, says Valorie Burton, life coach and author of *How Did I Get So Busy?* (Broadway) and other books about self-empowerment. "So many of us look to 'the next thing' to make us happy, and we forget to savor what's right in front of us," she reflects. "Happiness begins with noticing what there is to appreciate about your life at this moment." She recommends starting each day with an anticipation list of things to look forward to, and ending each evening by recalling three moments from the day that made you feel grateful—anything from a gorgeous sunrise to a loved one's smile. Practice sitting in quiet contemplation or prayer, Burton suggests. Then keep track of your blessings in a gratitude journal.

2} HANG OUT WITH JOYFUL PEOPLE. We need five positive interactions for every negative interaction in order for us to consider a relationship a happy one, psychologist John Gottman says. The point: Surround yourself with people who support and encourage you, and give a wide berth to those who criticize and deplete you. And be intentional in building strong bonds with others. "Social relationships are a powerful predictor of happiness, much more so than money," notes Daniel Gilbert in *Stumbling on Happiness* (Vintage). Indeed, a University of Illinois study showed that participants who reported the highest level of happiness also reported the strongest ties to friends and family members.

3} CHOOSE THE POSITIVE INTERPRETATION. "You're in charge of what things mean," says Carol Dweck, Ph.D., author of *Mindset: The New Psychology of Success* (Ballantine). "If your marriage fails, for example, you could make that mean that you're deficient as a human being and destined to be alone forever. Or you could decide there was something in the relationship that just didn't work. Does the latter mean you're unlovable? No. It could just mean that the other person wasn't the right partner for you."

> *"Don't wait around for other people to be happy for you. Any happiness you get, you've got to make yourself."* —ALICE WALKER

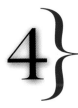

NOURISH BODY AND SOUL. Eat healthfully and get six to eight hours of sleep per night. And exercise regularly—the endorphin boost adds to your feeling of well-being and may help prevent diabetes, heart disease and other illnesses. Harvard lecturer Tal Ben-Shahar, Ph.D., adds: "Research shows that exercising three times a week for 30 minutes each session has the same effect as some of our most powerful drugs for alleviating depression." And give yourself permission to be human. "When we accept emotions such as fear, sadness and anxiety as natural, we are more able to overcome them," Ben-Shahar says.

Got Church?

A 2006 Pew Research report revealed that those who attend weekly services—of any faith—report feeling much happier than those who attend once a month or less.

GIVE—AND FORGIVE. Holding on to anger and resentment is an emotional weight that robs you of your joy. Let it go. "Happiness is spiritual peace—peace with God, with yourself and with others," explains A.R. Bernard, pastor and founder of New York's Christian Cultural Center and author of *Happiness Is...Simple Steps to a Life of Joy* (Touchstone Faith). And while you're handing out pardons, give away a few other things too: Generosity makes us feel as if we're making a difference by creating an environment of connection and love.

Your Pure Joy Playlist These songs can take you to your happy place.

"Soul II Soul's 'Keep on Movin' truly motivates."
—Lesette Heath, Alexandria VA

" 'Lovely Day' by Bill Withers makes me instantly think about my nieces."
—Bridgette Bartlett, Queens NY

" 'Let Go' by DeWayne Woods lets me know that with God, all things are possible."
—Nneka Garland, Sherman Oaks CA

"A sure fix to turn my day around is Natalie Cole's 'This Will Be (An Everlasting Love).' "
—Tresa Sanders, Cresskill NJ

"Instant joy: Marvin Gaye's 'Got to Give It Up' from his *Live at the London Palladium* album."
—Tamara Jeffries, Durham NC

"Sometimes you need a good booty-bumping song like 'Get Me Bodied' by Beyoncé."
—Nazenet Habtezghi, New York City

" 'Survivor' by Destiny's Child. The chorus makes me so happy because it reminds me this too shall pass."
—Maya Brooks, Atlanta

" 'Pretty Please (Love Me)' by Estelle always has me waving my arms and dancing."
—Cori Murray, New York City

"Bob Marley's 'Three Little Birds.' When he sings, 'Every little thing's gonna be alright,' I let go of whatever is vexing my spirit."
—Sharon Wynne, Queens NY

How Happy Are You?

Take this quiz to figure out your fulfillment factor.

1. On Monday morning, the first thing you see out of your bedroom window is a drenching downpour. Your first thought is...
A) It figures—I just had my hair done on Saturday.
B) Maybe it'll clear up by lunchtime.
C) Now I can wear my funky new rain boots!

2. A coworker can't wait to tell you about her promotion. You feel...
A) Envious. You've been angling in vain for a raise.
B) Heartened. It's good to work for a company that rewards from within.
C) Delighted. She works hard and deserves the step up.

3. You see your boyfriend talking with another woman. You...
A) Accuse him of cheating and break up with him in a vicious e-mail.
B) Act extra sweet next time you see him in the hope that he'll forget about her.
C) Assume she's a friend and go over to say hi.

4. You pray often because...
A) You hope the Lord will hear you one of these days.
B) It's the way you were raised.
C) You feel so blessed you just have to give thanks.

5. The jeans you were set to wear to a neighbor's barbecue refuse to zip. You decide to...
A) Stay home and order in.
B) Put on a different outfit and vow to start dieting—right after the barbecue, that is.
C) Throw on a skirt. Your legs look fabulous!

6. You've come up with a small-business idea, but you're finding it hard to attract investors. You...
A) Sulk. Clearly no one is interested because they think it's a stupid concept!
B) Forget it. You've got a decent job with good benefits; that's enough.
C) Tweak your business plan and try again. You have faith in your abilities to make this happen.

7. Your Friday night date cancels at the last minute. You...
A) Call your girlfriend and lament, "Why can't I find a guy who will treat me right?"
B) Ask him when next he thinks he will be available to see you.
C) Catch up with friends for a girls' night out and dance with a fine brother at the club. There's plenty of fish in the sea.

If You Answered...

Mostly A's,

YOU'RE POSTPONING JOY If your mindset hinges on "someday" happiness, you'll miss what's good and right in the moment. "Be open to the idea that life does not happen *to* you, but that life happens *for* you," says Robert Holden, Ph.D., author of *Happiness NOW!* (Hay House). And surround yourself with positive people. "Choose your 'flock' with intention," says Dallas professional business coach Beverly Alridge Wright. "Optimism—or the reverse—can be contagious." Remember that seeing yourself as a victim can be a self-fulfilling prophecy; visualize yourself a winner and you'll be one!

Mostly B's,

YOU'RE FAIRLY FULFILLED With your easygoing attitude, you appreciate what you have. Sometimes, though, you bend over backward to please others rather than taking charge of your own happiness. You tend to confuse contentment with complacency, settling when you might be striving. "Be willing to participate in your life more," Holden says. Setting goals for yourself is key. "Do something that gets the adrenaline flowing again and ignites your passion," suggests Wright. "Take an exercise or a dance class, or a community college course. Decide to try something new to make sure you are still growing."

Mostly C's,

YOU'RE SUPER SATISFIED "It's not that you've been spared life's challenges, but that you have chosen to see the upside of everything, demonstrating resilience and sunny optimism regardless of what life sends your way," says Wright. Mindful of your blessings, you consciously enjoy what you've got in the here and now. Continue to actively create your future, and you'll not only reap greater personal joy, but you'll also help make the planet a better place. "Your happiness is your gift to the world," says Holden. "People who follow their joy discover a depth of talent and creativity that inspires the world."

Is It More Than Just the Blues?

What depression feels like—and what to do when it hits. 》

What is depression?

Here's what it can sound like: *I can't fall asleep these days... I'll have a fourth slice of pie... I'm not in the mood for sex... Nothing really matters...* Major depression is a mental illness that affects your ability to function normally.

It can interfere with your ability to work, sleep, study, eat properly and enjoy life. Brain chemistry play a major role in depression, as do stress, genetics and environmental, psychological and social factors. Scientists are also exploring the influence of hormones, especially in women. With professional help, eighty percent of sufferers are able to successfully manage the condition.

Who gets it?

Depression is considered the number one cause of disability in women. Each year more than 19 million Americans experience a depressive episode, and 14 percent of Black women struggle with major depression at least once in their lifetime. Many more have contended with what experts call low-grade depression, which, if not addressed, could worsen. Among groups particularly at risk for mental illness— those who are homeless, incarcerated or exposed to violence—African-Americans tend to be overrepresented. Even single moms are more prone to

Signs of Depression If you experience five of these symptoms most days in a two-week period, you need to seek help, says Annelle Primm, M.D., M.P.H., director of the office of minority and national affairs at the American Psychiatric Association. Just have just one or two symptoms? Talk therapy may still be worth trying.

1. Sadness, anxiousness, or emptiness
2. Loss of interest in enjoyable activities and socializing
3. Change in sleeping (difficulty sleeping or sleeping too much)
4. Change in appetite (eating too much or too little)
5. Fatigue or a decrease in energy
6. Change in self-esteem (self-critical, feelings of guilt)
7. Hopelessness
8. Difficulty concentrating or making decisions
9. Thoughts of death or suicide

depression. A good partnership offers a level of protection against many stressors that can overwhelm a solo parent.

What are my options for handling it?

A thorough physician's assessment will determine your best approach. Some people with milder forms of depression respond well to therapy alone. Based on your symptoms, your doctor or psychiatrist may also prescribe medication. Alternative treatments such as acupuncture or herbal remedies may complement your treatment or even provide relief that traditional western medicine cannot.

Why are we hit harder?

Blacks with depression reported more severe impairment than Whites in a national survey. "People don't get the link between high rates of oppression and depression," says Brenda Wade, Ph.D., a San Francisco psychologist and author of *Power Choices: Signposts on Your Journey to Wholeness, Love, Joy and Peace* (Heartline Productions), "but there is the emotional legacy of racism." She explains that years of living under siege—with a body constantly churning out fight-or-flight hormones—can compromise the immune system of even the most resilient soul. Numerous studies also show clear links between depression and chronic diseases like heart disease, diabetes and obesity—diseases that affect Blacks in disproportionate numbers. Other factors: a lack of access to quality health care, a reluctance to seek help, misdiagnosis and inferior treatment compared with Whites.

Superwoman Syndrome

Beneath the gorgeous do and always-put-together ensemble, are you stressed and struggling? Too many of us never reach out for help because we fear others will consider us crazy or weak. "Black women have traditionally underrated their own needs," says Janet E. Taylor, M.D., an adult outpatient psychiatrist at Harlem Hospital. "We are so chronically sick and tired that's all we know."

Or perhaps you're the sister who snaps at her man and her kids? The one who gives shade to her coworkers? Some see you as troubled, but it's more likely you're depressed. "Black women don't often show depression as being sad or tired," says psychologist Brenda Wade. "Black women show depression through hyperirritability. Anger and rage feel better than depression."

Nobody is going to pull your Strong Black Woman Card or Superwoman cape if you admit you have "issues." Know that it takes strength to acknowledge that you need help and seek it out.

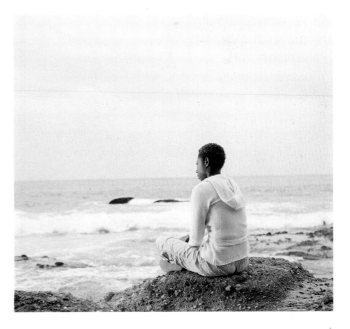

Take These Positive Steps Toward Healing

Get a checkup. Physical illnesses (such as thyroid problems and infections) can masquerade as depression. And if you're living with problems like multiple sclerosis, heart disease or HIV/AIDS, your mental distress could make your physical symptoms worse. Treating depression can help alleviate physical problems. Investigate your family history. Ask about the cousin who always seemed to make relatives antsy. "People's vulnerability to depression runs in the family," says Primm. That doesn't mean you'll get it, but it does cue you to pay attention.

Know you aren't being selfish. It's tough unlearning generational myths about being strong, selfless Black women. "People will take as much as you can give," says Taylor. "It's okay to put yourself first. This is about self-preservation."

Don't self-medicate. Turning to alcohol or illegal drugs to blunt the emotional pain of depression only exacerbates the problem and could add addiction to the mix.

Get the right support. Your primary care doctor or even your ob-gyn can refer you to mental health providers. Ask friends and relatives who've been in therapy; they might recommend the professionals they've worked with. Also check with your local hospitals and community clinics. If you want to see an African-American in particular, try referrals through The Association of Black Psychologists, abpsi.org/listing.htm or 202-722-0808.

5 Questions to Ask a Therapist

You may have to meet more than one to find a good fit. What to ask:

1. What experience do you have working with Black people?
The answer can offer important insights if the therapist is not African-American. "If they're defensive or dismissive, that's a red flag," says Kumea Shorter-Gooden, Ph.D., a licensed psychologist and systemwide director of international-multicultural initiatives at Alliant International University in Alhambra, California.

2. Tell me about your credentials and years of experience.
Licensing requirements vary by state, but a therapist should be licensed or supervised by someone who's licensed.

3. Do you have experience or expertise in _____?
Fill in the blank with issues you might be struggling with, such as sexual abuse, substance abuse, or relationship issues.

4. What is your therapy approach?
In psychoanalysis, you explore your past to figure out how it's affecting you now. Cognitive therapy focuses more on troubleshooting fears and anxieties right away. Expect to have homework and role playing with cognitive therapy.

5. Would you consider a lower fee?
Many therapists will adjust their fee based on what you can afford.

Prevention Prescription

Research shows that people who adopt a healthy lifestyle can keep depression at bay. "Many of the behaviors that are good for preventing heart disease, obesity and diabetes, are also good for preventing depression," says Primm. Here's what you can do:

1. **Exercise regularly.** Moving your body activates the feel-good hormones endorphins and dopamine, which are essentially "the body's own antidote to pain," Primm explains.

2. **Eat a balanced diet.** Avoid alcohol and excess sugar. A diet rich in B vitamins (found in whole grains, seafood, leafy greens and beans) is known to help ward off the effects of stress.

3. **Get enough sleep.** Experts say there is a link between sleep problems and depression. If you're not getting enough rest—aim for seven to eight hours a night—talk to your doctor. She can help you with lifestyle changes or write a prescription for a better night's sleep.

4. **Stay connected.** Beyond your social circle, stay active in your community. "Volunteer work contributes toward our own mental well-being," Primm says.

5. **Nurture your spirituality.** "It's not enough to focus on the physical, the emotional and the cognitive," Wade says, adding that "spirituality" goes beyond attending church and reading the Bible. "How do breakdowns become breakthroughs? Look for the lessons in your situation. What did you learn and how did you grow from your experience?"

6. **Talk about it.** "One thing that would help our community is if people said, 'I went to therapy,' or 'I'm in therapy,' " Shorter-Gooden says. "It would create more of a culture of acceptance and destigmatize the experience." If someone you know says she's in therapy, Shorter-Gooden says, tell her "That's wonderful that you're getting the help you deserve."

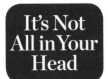

It's Not All in Your Head

"Science has shown a connection between what goes on in our environment and what goes on inside of us," Primm says, citing stressors such as living in socioeconomically disadvantaged neighborhoods. The excess noise and pollution, and higher likelihood of experiencing violence and crime, keep us continuously agitated and alert, and that 24/7 fight-or-flight response prompts our body to pump out neurochemicals such as norepinephrine and cortisol, which influence our mood and even our blood sugar. People with diabetes have a two-fold risk of experiencing depression compared with the general population. And people with depression have an increased risk of experiencing diabetes. While we can't always up and move to another neighborhood, we can intentionally create islands of calm in our lives.

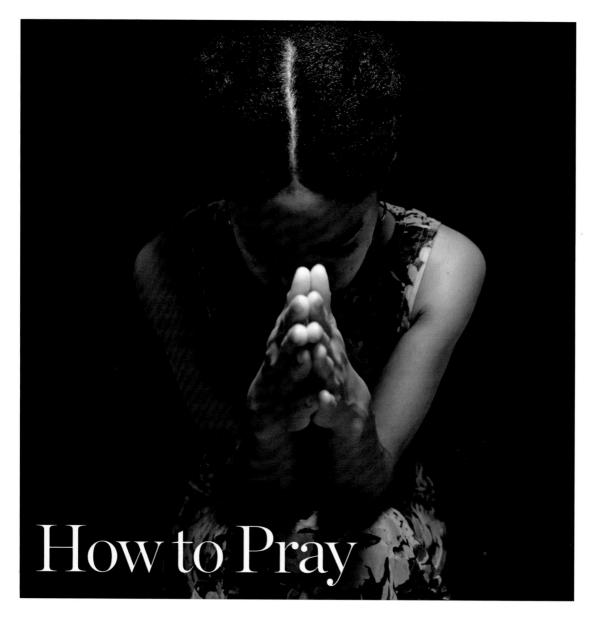

How to Pray

In her quest for a closer connection with God, Bonnie St. John talked to women she admired about the practice and power of prayer. Here, the motivational speaker and author of *How Strong Women Pray* (FaithWords) recalls the moving moments of faith others shared. 》

Pray All Day Prayer warriors talk to God upon waking, while taking a shower, driving to work, before meetings, as they prepare a meal. They pray through laughter and dancing, and by listening as well as speaking. Prayer isn't about asking for material things or giving God a to-do list. Prayer is simply taking the time to let God get close to us, so we don't miss out on our anointing.

Pray Out Loud There is power in shared prayer—when "two or more are gathered in His name." Join a prayer circle or try to attend church regularly. And pray out loud with your loved ones. To share such intimacy—your most private hopes, dreams and fears—can be scary and awkward at first, but in time you will begin to just talk about what is in your hearts, together before God.

Pray for Peace All prayers are answered by putting us in touch with God in some way. Once, when I was late for a meeting and whirling around the house, my 12-year-old daughter stopped me, put her hands on my shoulders and asked God that I be a source of peace, love and joy as I went out into the world. Her prayer completely changed my consciousness. The busier you are, the more you need to lean into prayer. The closeness you create with God will ripple out to bestow wisdom and serenity in every corner of your life.

Conversations With God
Strong women reveal how to pray with purpose

"Don't waste a lot of time praying for specific things. What you want may not be what God has in mind for you. Praying for courage and strength is the important thing."
—Dorothy Height, civil rights activist

"I sit in a quiet space with my eyes open, and I say whatever comes to heart."
—Vonetta Flowers, Olympic bobsled gold medalist

"You can't just reach out to God in a moment of need and then just go on with your life after the crisis passes. You have to stay connected to God, every morning and night."
—Immaculée Ilibagiza, Rwandan genocide survivor

"It is more effective to pray for God to work on me than it is for me to pray for God to work on other people."
—Johnnetta B. Cole, Ph.D., president emerita of Spelman and Bennett colleges

"If I could tell myself just one thing about prayer, I would tell myself to be even more grateful. I would like to be more grateful today than I was yesterday."
—Maya Angelou, poet and author

Quotes taken from *How Strong Women Pray* (FaithWords, 2007) by Bonnie St. John

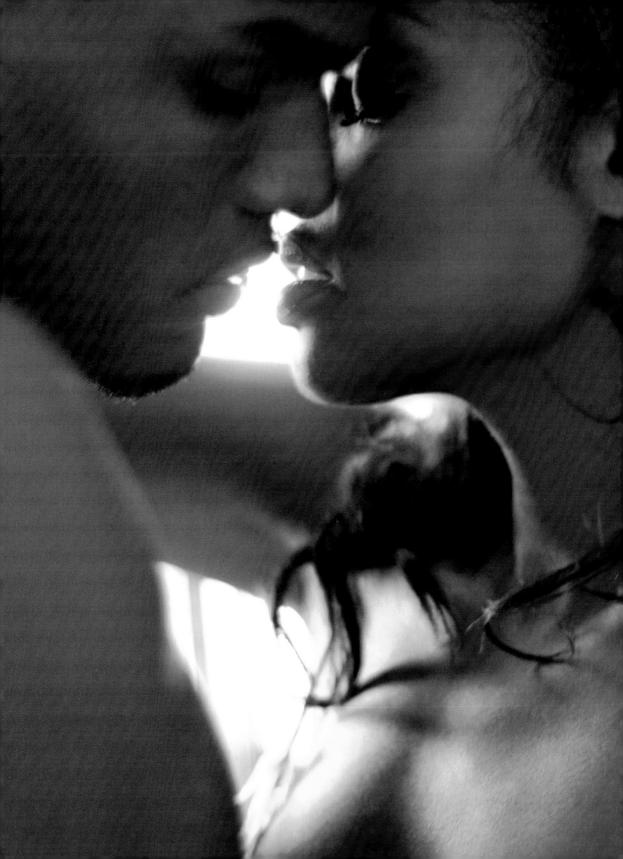

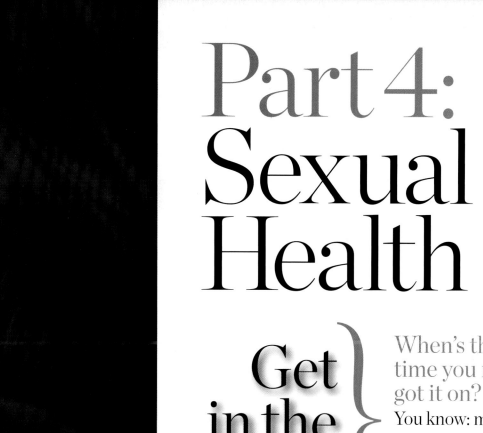

Part 4: Sexual Health

Get in the Mood

When's the last time you really got it on? You know: moaning, groaning, hanging on to the headboard, remember-it-and-sigh sex? To get there, you've got to make sure nothing ruins the moment, so we'll help you discover the reason behind your unpredictable period and the solution to that strange itch. You've also got to know what you want between the sheets and be comfortable asking for it. After all, good sex not only boosts your mood, it can strengthen your heart and immune system—not a bad way to double your pleasure. Jump right into all the intimate, expert-approved info you'll ever need. We promise, it'll be good for you. »

The Vagina Dialogues

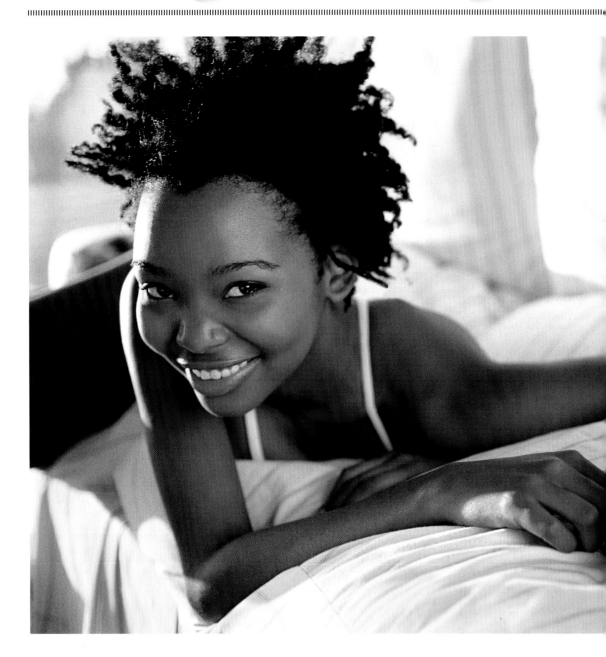

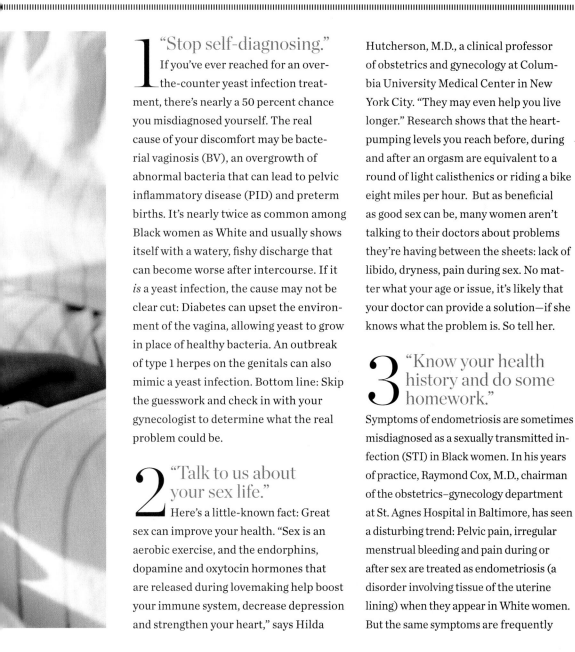

Intimate issues can have you frequently running to the doctor and sap your sex life. We got Black ob-gyns to give advice on stopping down-there drama before it starts. »

1 "Stop self-diagnosing."

If you've ever reached for an over-the-counter yeast infection treatment, there's nearly a 50 percent chance you misdiagnosed yourself. The real cause of your discomfort may be bacterial vaginosis (BV), an overgrowth of abnormal bacteria that can lead to pelvic inflammatory disease (PID) and preterm births. It's nearly twice as common among Black women as White and usually shows itself with a watery, fishy discharge that can become worse after intercourse. If it *is* a yeast infection, the cause may not be clear cut: Diabetes can upset the environment of the vagina, allowing yeast to grow in place of healthy bacteria. An outbreak of type 1 herpes on the genitals can also mimic a yeast infection. Bottom line: Skip the guesswork and check in with your gynecologist to determine what the real problem could be.

2 "Talk to us about your sex life."

Here's a little-known fact: Great sex can improve your health. "Sex is an aerobic exercise, and the endorphins, dopamine and oxytocin hormones that are released during lovemaking help boost your immune system, decrease depression and strengthen your heart," says Hilda Hutcherson, M.D., a clinical professor of obstetrics and gynecology at Columbia University Medical Center in New York City. "They may even help you live longer." Research shows that the heart-pumping levels you reach before, during and after an orgasm are equivalent to a round of light calisthenics or riding a bike eight miles per hour. But as beneficial as good sex can be, many women aren't talking to their doctors about problems they're having between the sheets: lack of libido, dryness, pain during sex. No matter what your age or issue, it's likely that your doctor can provide a solution—if she knows what the problem is. So tell her.

3 "Know your health history and do some homework."

Symptoms of endometriosis are sometimes misdiagnosed as a sexually transmitted infection (STI) in Black women. In his years of practice, Raymond Cox, M.D., chairman of the obstetrics–gynecology department at St. Agnes Hospital in Baltimore, has seen a disturbing trend: Pelvic pain, irregular menstrual bleeding and pain during or after sex are treated as endometriosis (a disorder involving tissue of the uterine lining) when they appear in White women. But the same symptoms are frequently treated as PID (an STI) in Black women. The conditions are commonly confused, especially among women with a history of infection. However, PID may be associated with a fever and foul-smelling discharge that you're not likely to have with endometriosis. Knowing the symptoms that set the two apart is the best way to ward off any in-office profiling.

4 "Ask for more than a Pap test."

Like a paper gown that doesn't close all the way and cold stirrups, certain things come standard on your ob-gyn visit. Pap smears are an annual event if you're 30 or younger. If you're over 30, however, you can have them every two to three years if you've had three consecutive negative tests or every three years if you've had both a Pap test and HPV test that came back negative. But that shouldn't be it. Chlamydia testing should be the norm for women under 26 because the disease runs rampant among young patients, is often asymptomatic and can damage the reproductive system. Mammograms should begin at age 40 but earlier if you have an immediate family member with breast cancer. Your M.D. should ask if you'd like an HIV test. And if you've been noticing a persistent white or grayish discharge, you may want to be tested for BV.

What's Your Period Trying to Tell You?

AN EXPERT DECODES YOUR MONTHLY VISIT. See your doctor to pinpoint specific issues and to address concerns.

PROBLEM: Heavy or lengthy menstruation

WHAT IT MEANS: Usually a hormonal imbalance or fibroids (noncancerous growths on the uterus) can result in periods that soak one or more tampons in an hour or last longer than a week. Other causes range from your birth control to endometrial cancer. "A heavy flow is serious and shouldn't be ignored," says Linda Bradley, M.D., director of Cleveland Clinic's Center for Menstrual Disorders, Fibroids and Hysteroscopic Services.

PROBLEM: Multiple visits during the month

WHAT IT MEANS: Stress or an overactive or underactive thyroid could be one reason you get your period more than once a month, but the most likely culprit is weight. "Women who are obese may have a hormonal imbalance that can lead to more frequent periods," Bradley explains.

PROBLEM: Missed period

WHAT IT MEANS: If pregnancy and menopause are out of the question, stress, being over- or underweight, or excessive exercise could be the reason. Simple lifestyle changes will likely get you back on track.

PROBLEM: Extreme pain or discomfort

WHAT IT MEANS: If a painkiller doesn't do the trick, you could have endometriosis (a condition in which tissue that usually grows inside the uterus grows outside of it) or fibroids. Ovarian cysts and even the use of an IUD have been found to cause pain as well.

[Do You Leak When You Laugh Know that urinary incontinence is reversible. This condition, which occurs in 47 percent of women ages 20 to 49, is sometimes preventable and always treatable. Ask your doctor for the best approach.]

Ob-Gyn Cheat Sheet:
Get More Out of Your Next Visit

What's on your mind?

Use this space to jot down two pressing issues to remember to bring up with your ob-gyn today—and don't be bashful.

1. _____

_____

_____

2. _____

_____

_____

What Your Doctor Wants to Know

Save time by having answers ready for these common questions:

1. When was your last period? Was there anything out of the ordinary?

2. Are you sexually active? Have you been tested for HIV in the past year? If not, do you want to be?

3. What type of birth control are you using, and how is it working?

4. Are you experiencing any pain? If so, how have you been treating it?

....

✳ **TIP:** Copy this page, fill it out, and take it to each appointment.

6 Questions for Your Ob-Gyn

1. Am I on the best birth control for me? There may be new options that would work better for you (like continuous birth control, the patch or Essure) or old methods you haven't considered (like an intrauterine contraceptive or the Sponge).

2. Should I get the HPV vaccine? Though HPV is extremely common, most women don't know the facts about this virus, which can cause genital warts and cervical cancer, or about the vaccine that has been shown to prevent some strains.

3. Can I have a prescription for the morning-after pill, just in case? You only have 72 hours to take it, so it's a good idea to get a prescription filled in advance to have on hand in case of an emergency.

4. Does my weight put me at risk for cancer? Overweight women are more susceptible to uterine and breast cancer, but ob-gyns don't often talk pounds with their patients unless asked. Here's a chance for you to start taking control of your weight.

5. Are mammograms my best option for detecting breast cancer? Due to their denser breasts, young Black women may want to ask their doctors if an ultrasound or an MRI may be a better option.

6. Can I get an HIV test here?

Safe Sex 101

Whether you're single or married or casually dating, you need to be aware and be safe. Black women have been hardest hit by sexually transmitted infections (STIs). The leading cause of death for Black women ages 25 to 34 is HIV/AIDS. We're also at the highest risk for herpes, and we're seven times more likely to contract chlamydia than White women. If you're not using condoms—every time—this quiz will convince you otherwise. »

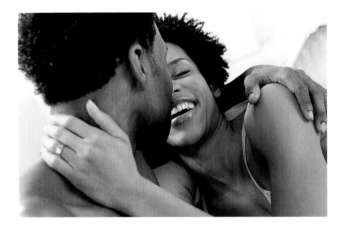

Q That fine man you've been dating is giving you the please-baby-please speech but says he doesn't use condoms. You decide to have mutual unprotected oral sex. After all, that's much safer than condom-free vaginal sex, isn't it? TRUE or FALSE

A FALSE. "Oral sex is often considered problem-free, but the fact is you can still transmit herpes, gonorrhea and other sexually transmitted diseases and infections," explains Aimee R. Kreimer, Ph.D., an epidemiologist at the National Cancer Institute. And add the human papilloma virus (HPV), long linked to cervical cancer, to that list. A study coauthored by Kreimer found that oral HPV infection is a strong risk factor in the development of throat cancer. For oral sex, you should use barrier methods—that means a condom on him, and dental dam on you.

Q You got herpes in college, but you haven't had symptoms in years. Are you clear to have unprotected sex? YES or NO

A NO. "Once you've been diagnosed with herpes, you're still at risk for recurrent episodes and able to infect others," says Kimberly D. Gregory, M.D., an associate professor at the University of California at Los Angeles and vice-chair of obstetrics at Cedars-Sinai Medical Center. Avoid sex if you have symptoms. Tell your partner about your condition, and use barrier methods to decrease the chances of transmission.

Q You're getting ready to go out with your guy and you just might get your groove on. If you put in a female condom before you go out, can you leave it there for later? YES or NO

A YES. "Female condoms really put you in a position of power," says Renee Beaman, R.N., executive director of the Bethel A.M.E. Church's Beautiful Gate Outreach Center in Wilmington, Delaware. Just don't leave one in for more than eight hours. And practice inserting and removing them a few times before wearing one during sex. "They can be tricky to put in," Beaman says.

Q You run into your ex one weekend. Caught in the rapture, you end up having unprotected sex with him. No worries— you can rule out HIV by getting tested for the virus on Monday. TRUE or FALSE

A FALSE. Beaman sees so many panicky people request HIV tests after a wild weekend that she's dubbed the phenomenon Manic Mondays. "But it takes three months before there are enough antibodies in your system to test for HIV," she says, "so if you've just engaged in high-risk behavior, you're going to have to wait 90 days to know your status."

FACT: One quarter of people who have HIV don't know they're infected.

HIV+AIDS:
What's the Difference?

Many people think HIV and AIDS are the same thing. Here's what's what: You can contract HIV (Human Immunodeficiency Virus) through the exchange of semen, vaginal fluid and blood, but it doesn't mean that you have AIDS (Acquired Immunodeficiency Syndrome). Doctors consider an HIV-positive person to have AIDS only after the virus has worn down his or her immune system so much that he or she becomes vulnerable to opportunistic infections, such as pneumonia.

Get Tested for HIV

Your private physician can do the test, or you can visit a free low-cost clinic in your area. Go to hivtest.org and enter your zip code to find places that perform testing.

Q Your doctor just told you that you have HPV. She suggests you tell your previous partners. If the man you just broke up with didn't have any warts, could he still have the virus? YES or NO

A YES. "HPV is often a silent disease, especially in men," Gregory says. "He could still have and spread the virus even though he doesn't have any signs." According to the Centers for Disease Control and Prevention, about half of sexually active men and women will contract HPV in their lifetimes. Unfortunately, there's no HPV test for men (although there is treatment for genital warts), but your ex should know he's been exposed so he can take precautions.

The ABCs of STIs

STI	WHAT IT IS
Chlamydia	This bacterial infection is the number one reported sexually transmitted infection (STI) in America, with an estimated 2.8 million new cases each year. It often presents no symptoms, though some women may experience an abnormal vaginal discharge or burning during urination, lower abdominal and back pain, nausea, fever, pain during intercourse or bleeding. Left untreated, chlamydia can cause pelvic inflammatory disease (PID), which may lead to infertility or ectopic pregnancy.
Genital Herpes	A shocking one in two African-Americans is infected with genital herpes, which is caused by herpes simplex virus Type 1 (HSV-1) and Type 2 (HSV-2). Both strains can be transmitted during sexual contact by sores the virus causes, as well as between outbreaks. An HSV-1 infection typically causes fever blisters that are spread by kissing or oral sex. An HSV-2 infection can cause blisters on or around the genitals or rectum that break leaving very painful sores, and flulike symptoms.
Gonorrhea	More than 350,000 cases of this bacterial infection were reported in 2006. It's usually spread during sexual contact and sometimes from mother to baby during delivery. Gonorrhea is often asymptomatic, but can cause burning during urination, increased vaginal discharge that may be yellow and thick, or vaginal bleeding between periods. Like chlamydia, untreated gonorrheal infections can lead to PID, ectopic pregnancy and infertility. Gonorrhea can be life-threatening if it infects the joints.
HIV/AIDS	Black women account for 64 percent of new HIV infections among women. The only way to know if you are infected is to be tested. Untreated, HIV leaves the body vulnerable to a host of infections, from tuberculosis and rare skin cancers to unusual forms of pneumonia. HIV attacks the immune system's white blood cells called T cells or CD4 cells. When the virus weakens immunity to the point that the body succumbs to specific types of infections and has a low number of T cells, a person has AIDS.
Human Papilloma Virus (HPV)	A sexually active person will likely get HPV at some point in his or her life. As many as 20 million Americans are thought to have genital HPV, with an estimated 6.2 million more infected every year. Most people think that vaginal warts put them at risk for cancer, but it's the strain of infection that does not cause warts that appears to be the high-risk form of HPV. Some strains of HPV, left unchecked, have been shown to cause cervical cancer.

Need a refresher course on sexually transmitted infections? Our rundown shows you what you're risking when you have unprotected sex. 》

HOW DO I TREAT IT?	HOW DO I PROTECT MYSELF?
See your doctor for antibiotics. A single dose of azithromycin or one week of doxycycline (twice daily) are the most common treatments. Your partner will need treatment, too.	Use condoms or a dental dam.
Genital herpes can be managed with antiviral drugs such as Valtrex, Famvir and Zovirax, but no cure exists.	It can be transmitted even when a person doesn't show signs. Ask your partner if he has herpes before having protected sex.
"Only one drug class remains for treating gonorrhea: cephalosporins," says Stuart M. Berman, M.D., chief of the epidemiology and surveillance branch in the division of STD Prevention at the Centers for Disease Control in Atlanta.	With gonorrhea becoming increasingly resistant to traditional drug treaments, it's critical that you use condoms or a dental dam.
There is no cure for HIV, but with recent breakthroughs in antiretroviral treatments, early detection makes an enormous difference in the length and quality of life for a person with HIV.	Using condoms or a dental dam can prevent the sexual transmission of HIV.
Get regular Pap smears and HPV tests. And look into the groundbreaking HPV vaccine, Gardasil, which may protect women up to age 45 against four strains of the virus (and thus cervical cancer).	HPV is passed on by contact with uncovered body parts, so use protection and talk to your partner about his sexual health.

Condom Talk: Five Easy Comebacks

Gina Wingood, Sc.D., M.P.H., suggests these smart responses when he's trying to convince you to go bare.

He says: "You're on the pill, so we're okay."
You say: "I like to use a condom anyway to protect us from infections we may not realize we have."

He says: "I'll probably lose my erection."
You say: "Not if I do it!"

He says: "You think I'm some kind of player?"
You say: "No, but it's best to use a condom."

He says: "A real man doesn't use them."
You say: "A real man cares about the woman and their relationship."

He says: "I won't have sex if I have to use one."
You say: "So let's put it off until we can agree."

Fibroids

Up to 80 percent of Black women will have them by the time they reach age 60. Get a handle on this health problem and learn how to overcome it here. »

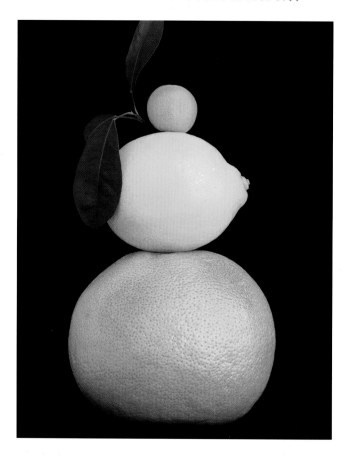

What are fibroids?

Fibroids are usually noncancerous tumors that can appear inside, on the outer surface, or within the walls of your uterus.

What does having fibroids feel like?

Fibroids can be as tiny as the eraser on your pencil or as large as a grapefruit. You may not notice them at all, or they could cause heavy periods, pelvic pressure or pain, a bloated abdomen, trouble getting pregnant and miscarriages. In African-American women, these growths tend to develop at an earlier age and to have more severe effects than in women from other ethnic groups.

Why are we affected more severely?

Genetics appears to influence whether or not some women will develop the condition. Our size may also be a factor: "Obesity may directly influence the development of larger bulk tumors," says Margaret Larkins-Pettigrew, M.D., an assistant professor of ob-gyn and reproductive sciences at the University of Pittsburgh.

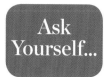

Ask Yourself...

DOES MY DIET PUT ME AT RISK? Some experts tell their patients to avoid food with hormones in them (like certain meats and cow's milk). But while diet appears to be related to the risk of developing fibroids, experts say, there is no evidence that changing your diet will change the symptoms of fibroids or the progression of disease.

Treating Fibroids
What approach might work best for you?

Myomectomy

What it is: The surgical removal of fibroids, leaving the uterus intact. Surgery can be done vaginally, laparoscopically or through an abdominal incision. Fertility may be maintained.
Consider: General or regional anesthesia and a hospital stay are required. Fibroids may eventually recur, and complications such as urinary-tract infections, though rare, do occur.
Recommended for: Women trying to maintain their fertility.

Uterine Artery Embolization

What it is: Sand-size particles are put into the uterine artery to permanently block the blood supply that feeds fibroids. With less blood traveling to them, fibroids become smaller.
Consider: Typically, a one-night hospital stay is needed for pain management. Fertility may be compromised, and new fibroids can emerge. Early menopause may also occur.
Recommended for: Women with several small and medium-size fibroids and patients who are obese, have uncontrolled diabetes, or might not be good candidates for general anesthesia. The procedure is generally not suggested for women who want to have children.

MR-guided Focused Ultrasound Surgery

What it is: The ExAblate 2000 system uses MRI technology to see, and ultrasound waves to destroy fibroids. It's an outpatient procedure; general anesthesia is not needed. Women can resume normal activity in a day, but fertility may or may not be preserved.
Consider: Not for the claustrophobic because you're placed in an MRI tube, sedated but awake, for up to four hours. Catheterization is required.
Recommended for: Women with no more than six fibroids of a specified size (two to ten centimeters), due to limitations on the amount of time you can spend in an MRI tube.

Hysterectomy

What it is: Surgical removal of the uterus; the uterus and cervix; or the uterus, cervix and ovaries. Surgery is done vaginally or through the abdomen. Fibroids do not recur.
Consider: General or regional anesthesia is necessary, and there is a long recovery period, usually about six weeks. Severely obese women or those with other medical conditions such as uncontrolled diabetes might be at higher risk for complications. If ovaries are removed before menopause has occurred, early menopause is likely.
Recommended for: Women who have completed child bearing, experience severe symptoms such a bleeding, and have serious problems with the size and number of their fibroids.

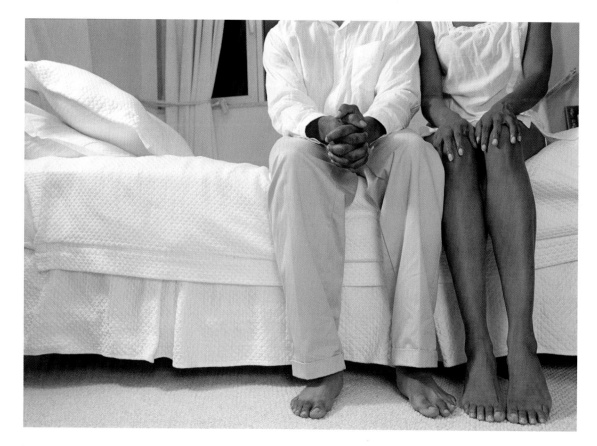

Your Most Intimate Questions, Answered

Nothing's too weird—or too wild—for Hilda Hutcherson, M.D., our sexpert, a clinical professor of obstetrics and gynecology at Columbia University Medical Center in New York City and author of *Pleasure: A Woman's Guide to Getting the Sex You Want, Need and Deserve* (Perigee Trade). Here, some of her best advice for happy lovemaking. »

I give my husband oral sex every time we make love, but he never returns the favor. How do I get him to go down on me?

Just ask for what you want! Men adore *getting* **oral sex.** While you're doing all the work, he can lie back and enjoy himself. Likewise, women love receiving oral sex. It's one of the few times you can focus only on the wonderful sensations alone. In fact, it's one of the easiest ways for many women to experience orgasm.

Sex should be mutually enjoyable, and both of you should do everything to help the other receive the greatest possible pleasure. The key is communication. Have a conversation about what's working in your sex life and what's not. Let your man know how much you want to experience oral sex. It's likely that he'll oblige. If he's reluctant, offer to help allay any apprehensions he might have. If he's still disinclined, withhold fellatio until he changes his mind. Bet he will.

···

My boyfriend talks a little too dirty during sex. How can I get him to tone it down?

Erotic exchanges can be a sensual way to communicate your desires while providing the spark you need to increase passion and pleasure. But sex talk needs to be comfortable and arousing for *both* partners. And while racy words can serve as an aphrodisiac for some, they can cause others to cringe with embarrassment.

Asking your man to stop talking completely may rob him of some of the pleasure he receives during sex. Instead, try to meet him halfway. Take a turn talking dirty to him, but only as far as you feel acceptable. Read an erotic story or watch a X-rated movie, and note the phrases you find arousing. When making love, say the kind of words you'd prefer he say to you. He'll take the hint. If he doesn't, ask him to lighten it up a bit. Just remember: Have the conversation when you're not having sex, and you're both relaxed.

···

I have three children, work full-time, and attend college part-time. I'm exhausted, and most days I have no sex drive. How can I get back the great love life my husband and I once had?

It's no wonder that you have no energy or sexual desire. After the kids, the home, the job and schoolwork, sex can seem like just one more thing you have to do for someone else. But intimacy—both emotional and physical—is essential for a healthy marriage. When you have sex, you and your husband produce several chemicals. One, oxytocin, is thought to increase bonding in couples. Satisfying sex also has other benefits, like relieving stress and improving sleep. Therefore you must make lovemaking a priority and carve out time for it. Here are some ways to make that happen:

❋ Schedule sexual "dates" with your husband. The anticipation will boost your libido. Pick a day and time every week for sex, and try to stick to it. Let a babysitter or relative take care of the children so you and your man can spend time together uninterrupted.

* Have sex first thing in the morning. Or ask your husband to take care of the kids and evening chores while you nap before a night of lovemaking. Great sex requires energy.
* Add toys, erotica and fantasy or change the location of your sex play to keep things fresh and desirable. Even checking in to a hotel for a night may add an extra spark.

My boyfriend's penis is so big that neither he nor I can enjoy sex. How can we make our sexual relationship better?

Many women think that bigger is better. Others, find sex with a well-endowed man to be uncomfortable, even painful. If properly aroused and relaxed, your vagina can accommodate any size penis. The key is finding creative ways to make sex more pleasurable.

To help you relax, begin with a warm bath and an erotic massage by your partner. Spend time on foreplay. It increases blood flow to the vagina, making it become longer, wider and more moist. Insertion is also easier if he wears a lubricated latex condom or when you apply an ample amount of water-based lubricant to your vagina and his penis. While making love, choose a position in which you can guide the thrusting, such as woman on top, or one that prevents deep insertion, like lying face to face. And remember, oral sex and manual stimulation may be just as satisfying as intercourse.

I've been experiencing vaginal dryness for a month now, and sex has become unbearable. Could this be a sign of a more serious health problem? And are there natural remedies I could turn to?

Lubrication of your vagina signals sexual arousal. But sometimes you don't produce enough moisture. And when two dry surfaces rub against each other, they produce friction and heat. Your vagina swells, and sex becomes painful. Taking certain medications, including birth control pills and antihistamines, can leave your vagina dry. Chronic medical problems like diabetes and infections as well as stress, douching and smoking can lead to vaginal dryness. A drop in the production of estrogen as we age can cause blood flow to the vagina to decrease and also limit lubrication. To get your juices flowing, try these tactics:

* Spend lots of time on foreplay. Women generally need more time to become aroused than men, and this difference increases as we get older. Don't allow yourself to be rushed into sex before you are wet and ready.
* Try lubricants. They increase vaginal moisture and can also add spice to your sex life. Introduce them during foreplay. For added excitement try flavored or warming lubricants that can be purchased at an adult shop or online.
* Apply vitamin E oil to your vaginal tissue several times a week (but avoid other oils like Vaseline—they may remain in your vagina and increase your risk of infections). Both vitamin E oil and Vaseline can degrade a condom, so don't use either during intercourse.

I assumed it was easy for men to orgasm. But my husband takes too long to climax, and I find myself tired, frustrated and sore. What am I doing wrong? How can I speed him up?

While some men will reach an orgasm after a few minutes, others require 30 minutes or more. Some, concerned about pleasing their partners, have perfected methods to delay their ejaculation. It's possible that your husband is trying to give you the prolonged stimulation he thinks you need. He may be relieved to hear that it's not necessary.

It's also possible that he has delayed ejaculation, which makes it difficult for him to reach orgasm during sex. There may be psychological or physical reasons for this problem. Men who grew up in a home where sex was considered dirty or sinful, or those who fear pregnancy or STIs, may find it difficult to let go during sex. Also, medical problems like diabetes, high blood pressure and alcohol abuse and such medications as antidepressants can also delay orgasm.

You're not doing anything wrong and shouldn't doubt your sexual adequacy. Let him know you love having sex with him, but it's hard to participate in prolonged intercourse without becoming sore. Use oral sex, manual stimulation or even a vibrator to bring him close to an orgasm prior to intercourse. Use lubricants to keep your vagina from becoming dry, and choose positions that give him more stimulation, such as man on top.

An Even Better Climax

Yes, an orgasm is an involuntary muscle contraction. But there's plenty you can do to control and enhance it. Here, four ways to get started tonight.

Free your mind. Orgasms begin in the brain and require a fair amount of concentration. So eliminate climax-killers like your beeping Blackberry and negative thoughts about your thighs and focus on feeling sexy.

Know what works. Close your eyes and think back to that passage from a romantic book that you read twice, a leg-crossing steamy movie scene, or the best orgasm you ever had. Figure out what about those moments drove your body wild so you can repeat it in your mind or with your man.

Switch things up. Imagine eating your favorite meal every single day. That could start to dull your palate, right? Same goes for sex. If you've got a favorite sex toy or position, consider trying a new one. Your body could get used to having the same type of stimuation every time—lowering your sexual horizons.

Get into position. When you're on top during intercourse, the combination of deep penetration and clitoral stimulation is more intense than in any other position. You direct how the penis is stimulating you, so your orgasm chances are increased.

Sexy at Every Age

20s }

You should have started annual gynecological exams as soon as you turned 18 or became sexually active. You're at your most fertile now, and because you're more likely to experiment and take risks, you're also more likely to contract an STI (sexually transmitted infection).

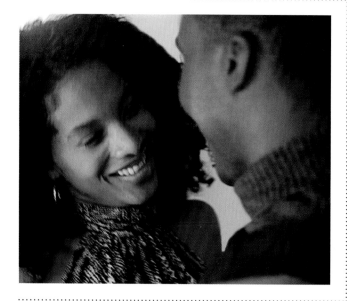

Say What Feels Good

Younger women need to tell their partners what stimulates them sexually, says Gloria Richard-Davis, M.D., chair of Ob-Gyn at Meharry Medical College. Don't be too embarrassed to speak up!

Tell Your Doctor

If your sexual activities have increased your risk of disease, let your doctor know so she can do a screening beyond the routine breast exam, Pap smear, HPV (human papillomavirus) screening and chlamydia test.

Practice Safe Sex

Two thirds of STIs occur in people 25 and younger, and women are more likely to be infected than men. Many STIs have no signs or symptoms but can do serious damage to your reproductive organs. How to protect yourself? Either don't have sex or use barrier contraception—every time. Purchase and carry condoms yourself.

Get the Right Birth Control

You'll want contraception that fits your body and your budget. The Pill is popular among women in their 20s, but some say it lowers libido. Keep trying until you find the method that suits you.

Glove Love

Make safe sex sensational by venturing to condomania.com for textured, rainbow colored and vibrating condoms. Just remember it's the latex and polyurethane ones that protect you from STIs.

You can be sensual and sexually vibrant no matter what your number. Here's what you should consider in your 20s, 30s, 40s, 50s and beyond. »

30s }

You may be settling down and starting to plan your family now. The security of having a stable, committed relationship may enable you to become more sexually adventurous, but balancing career responsibilities and babies once they arrive, can leave you feeling not in the mood.

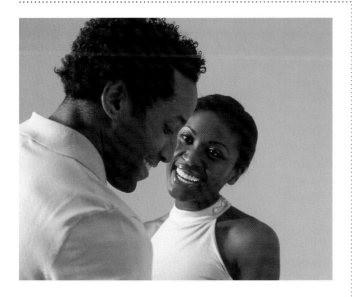

Create Intimacy
You're more confident with your body and willing to express your needs. Remind him that as much as you adore him, for most women, good sex becomes sensational when you and your partner are emotionally in tune.

Get Your Annual Exam
Some MDs recommend getting a baseline mammogram at 35 and digital breast exams, which are better at reading denser breast tissue (common among young women). Routine chlamydia screenings is also a good idea.

Better Safe Than Sorry
Want an exclusive sexual relationship? Make sure your man knows that—and agrees to it. "Just because you're monogamous doesn't mean your partner is," says Gloria Richard-Davis, M.D. If you have a hunch that he's sexually active with someone other than you, then go with your gut and protect yourself.

Listen to Your Clock
"In your 30s you start to see a gradual decline in fertility," Richard-Davis says. If you're under 35 and have failed to become pregnant after trying for six months, start exploring fertility issues with your doctor.

Make It fast
Sex doesn't have to be a ten-hour tantric affair. Multitask with your man in the shower or have a quickie in between the sheets when you're tired. The important thing is to just connect with each other.

40s }

If you're trying to conceive, know that your chances decline significantly in this decade. You might also experience the low libido, irregular periods and sweats of perimenopause. As for sexual satisfaction, you know what you want. Now you just need time and energy to get yours.

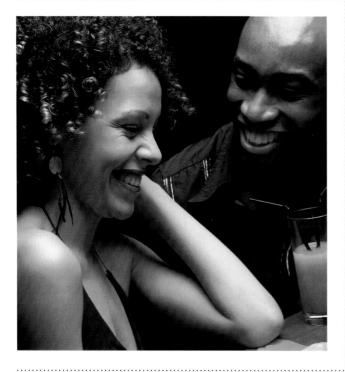

Consider Fertility Issues
Women trying to conceive at this age may be struggling with conditions that affect their fertility, such as fibroids, Richard-Davis says. If you're perimenopausal and don't want to get pregnant, continue to use birth control until you've missed periods for 12 months.

Know What Satisfies
You're at ease with your body—whatever shape it's in. But perimenopause could affect your sexual desire, and lower estrogen levels mean less lubrication in the vagina. Talk to your partner about your needs, and use lubricants and toys to keep sex enjoyable.

Do "The Exercise"
Try Kegel exercises to strengthen your pubococcygeal muscle to forestall loss of tissue tone that can contribute to urinary incontinence: Squeeze your pelvic-floor muscle as if you're trying to stop urination. Not only will that help "hold it" when you've got to go or when you sneeze, but it also guarantees more pleasure during sex. And remember, if you're not in an exclusive monogamous relationship, continue to use barrier protection.

Be Proactive About Care
Starting at age 40, annual mammograms are a must. One in eight women develops breast cancer, and Black women also die disproportionately because they're diagnosed at a more advanced stage and they're vulnerable to more aggressive forms of the disease.

Pleasure Principle
Am I taking too long? Will this get me pregnant? Self-conscious thoughts can kill the passion. Try fantasizing during sex—even if it's about someone else—so you can focus in on pleasure.

50s

With menopause, your ovaries stop releasing eggs and estrogen, so you'll have no worries about getting pregnant. Some women enjoy this new sexual freedom and experience a boost in libido, while others struggle with weight gain, moodiness and low sex drive.

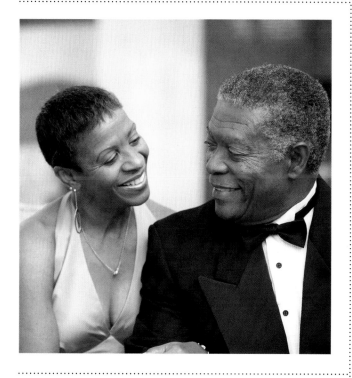

Manage Menopause

Up to 90 percent of women experience significant menopausal symptoms in their fifties. The most common: hot flashes and night sweats. Your doc might prescribe hormone therapy or antidepressants (though they can decrease libido) to control flashes.

Try Something New

You're confident of your body. But after years of the same old thing with the same old partner, you might want a new thrill. Experiment in different locations with sex toys and masturbation. As long as you're not hurting anybody, you and your partner can do what works for you.

Use a Condom

Doctors are seeing more older women coming in with herpes, HPV and HIV. (Almost 10 percent of AIDS cases in American women occur in women over 50.) That's because older women are less likely to use a condom. Often they are recently divorced and just returning to the dating scene. "Just because you're mature, don't assume your partner is too," says Richard-Davis. "I tell older women the same thing I tell my teenagers: Don't get lost in the moment!"

Stay Physically Strong

In addition to your pelvic, Pap and mammogram, you should have bone-density testing, experts say. You're at greater risk for osteoporosis and hip fractures now. Regular exercise and a diet rich in calcium and Vitamin D are keys to continued strength and vitality.

Spice It Up

Want to pepper up your sex life? Try a strip tease. Slowly peel off your clothes, tossing each piece to him in an exaggerated fashion. Keep it fun and carefree, and most of all, remember to laugh!

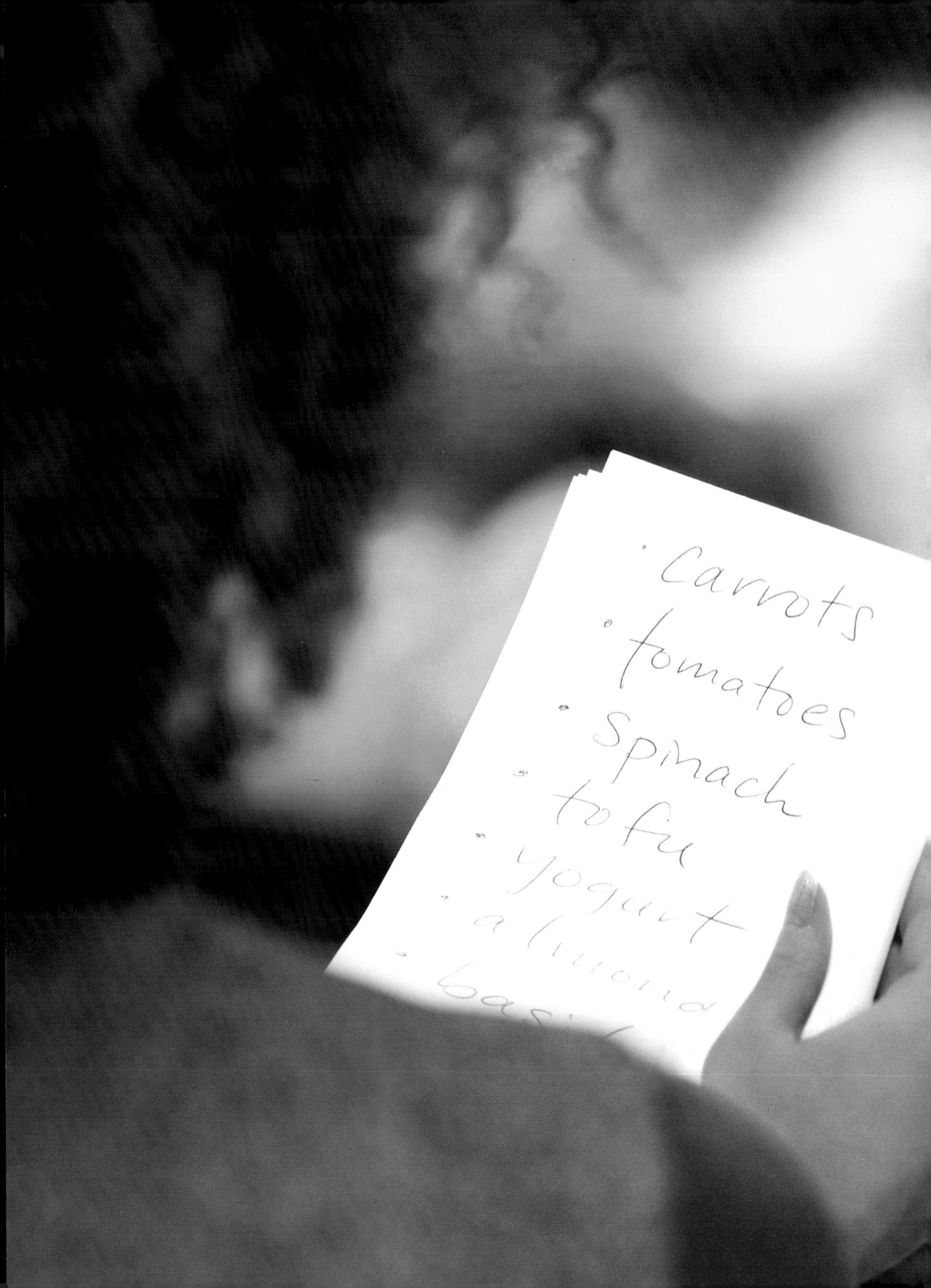
carrots
tomatoes
spinach
tofu
yogurt

Part 5: Healthy Food Fast

Good Food Is Your Friend

Here's what healthful eating is: It's feeding your hunger and your other senses as well—enjoying the sweet-spicy aroma of jerk-seasoned turkey burgers, the red-red of a watermelon wedge, the tang of pickle relish, mustard and celery in your favorite potato salad. It's about giving and sharing meals with friends and family, and getting in touch with your own body's nutritional needs. Here's what healthful eating is not: It's not about starving yourself or serving up food that tastes like twigs and Styrofoam. And it's not about judgment or denial. In this section, to celebrate heathful eating, we bring you three weeks of mouthwatering meals, recipes just like your Mama used to make—only easier on the calories, fat and salt. We also serve up a portion-savvy food guide, power breakfasts, energizing snacks and guilt-free desserts. You'll find that yes, you can have your cake and eat it too. »

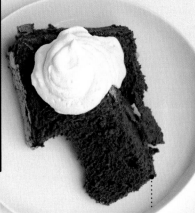

[Nutrition experts say this is how most folks typically fix a meal. »

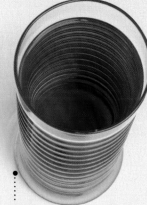

JUST DESSERTS

A large slice, no fruit and scoop of ice cream take this treat over the top.

GET YOUR DRINK ON

Oversize tumblers can trick you into drinking more than your 8-ounce serving.

Servin' It Up!

It's not only what you eat but how much. Experts size up proper portions to save you calories. »

GRAINS/STARCH

We tend to load up on high-calorie and high-fat sides while also doubling up on starch portions.

PROTEIN

When it comes to meat, we often pile on up to three times (10 to 12 ounces) what we need.

VEGETABLE

We think we're doing well by squeezing in a few string beans or a floret of broccoli.

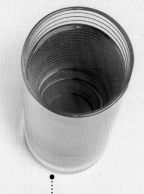

DESERT DONE RIGHT

Take a narrow slice. "And fill up on fruit," says Lisa R. Young, Ph.D., R.D., an adjunct professor of nutrition at New York University and author of *The Portion Teller Plan* (Broadway). "Eat up, but when you feel full, stop."

GRAINS/STARCH

Should take up ¼ of a regular-size dinner plate. Think one cup or a portion the size of a fist or a tennis ball.

PROTEIN

Three to four ounces or ¼ of your plate. "Think deck of cards, or the palm of your hand," says Young. For fish, think the size of a checkbook.

GET YOUR DRINK ON

Put your beverage in an 8-ounce glass: "A glass that's full looks filling," says Jonny Bowden, Ph.D., C.N.S., board-certified nutrition specialist and author of *The Most Effective Natural Cures on Earth* (Fair Winds Press).

VEGETABLE

"This is your biggest portion," says Bowden. Veggies should comprise ½ of your meal. You can eat as much of nonstarch vegetables (no potato, corn, squash or peas) as you want, as long as they're prepared healthfully.

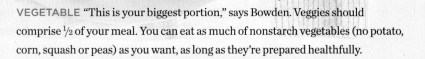

Foods That Energize

For more pep, great skin and sizzling sex, stock up on these power foods.

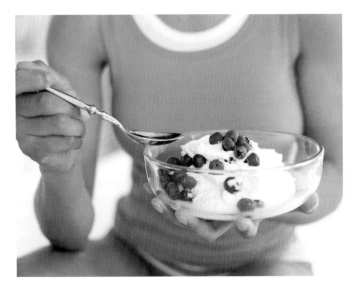

»Yogurt

Yogurt with live bacteria called probiotics bolsters the body's ability to fight infections and helps the intestines absorb more nutrients from food. The same bacteria can make yogurt easier to digest by those with lactose intolerance, while the dose of vitamin B12 is an energy booster. With its bone-strengthening calcium, yogurt is excellent for growing bones, and in older women, helps prevent osteoporosis. Try to eat one cup a day. Choose brands with live active cultures and opt for the lowest fat content.

⌃ Blueberries

Just one cup is loaded with 21 grams of energy-boosting carbohydrates, nearly four grams of appetite-suppressing fiber and 14 milligrams of vitamin C—all for just 83 calories. The substance that gives them their distinctive hue, anthocyanin, helps protect cells from damage that can lead to certain cancers, heart disease, varicose veins and urinary tract infections. One-half to 1-cup a day helps meet the recommended daily allowance of two cups of fruit. Blackberries, purple grapes, plums and raisins offer similar benefits. Fresh or flash-frozen, sprinkle them in your cereal, add them to plain low- or no-fat yogurt, or toss them in a blender with yogurt or low-fat milk and a little honey and ice for a delicious smoothie.

»Salmon

Fish is low in calories and saturated fat and an excellent source of lean protein. The cold-water varieties, such as salmon (and sardine and mackerel), are also rich in omega-3 fatty acids, which protect against heart disease and help fight depression. Try to eat a 3-to-4-ounce serving two to three times a week. When possible, opt for wild Alaskan over other varieties, since it is less likely to contain dangerous pollutants than farm-raised fish. Or use canned salmon; the bones add calcium.

When you hit that midafternoon slump, it's so easy to reach for a sugary pick-me-up. But there are smarter options. We asked nutritionists Constance Brown-Riggs, R.D., and Rovenia Brock, Ph.D., for tips on the best foods to boost energy, calm nerves and improve overall well-being. »

»Almonds

A great protein snack, almonds are an excellent source of zinc, which contibutes to smooth, unblemished skin. They're also high in magnesium and fiber—two proven energy boosters, particularly useful in fueling your workout routine. Limit your serving to 20 almonds (they're packed with calories). Buy individual serving sizes or dispense a serving in a baggie and drop them in your purse for an on-the-go snack. You can also use them to top salads or cereal.

» Collard Greens

Collard greens are a low-calorie, high-impact food. One cup of cooked greens has just 49 calories, and is an excellent source of vitamin C, disease-fighting antioxidants, and folate, an essential vitamin for expectant moms. Collards and other leafy green vegetables, such as spinach, turnip greens and kale, are also good sources of magnesium, which may help reduce water retention. Try to eat one cup of collards three times a week, but don't cook them in bacon fat or ham hocks, which negates the benefits.

»Sweet Potatoes

Low in fat and high in fiber and antioxidants, sweet potatoes have twice the recommended daily allowance of vitamin A, which keeps skin from becoming dry. They're also loaded with complex carbohydrates, so they keep you feeling fuller longer. Brown-Riggs recommends three cups a week, but diabetics and people who are overweight should limit themselves to a half cup a week. Like pumpkin, acorn and butternut squash, sweet potatoes taste great baked with a bit of cinnamon sprinkled on top.

»Black Beans

Packed with soluble fiber that provides steady, slow-burning fuel and plenty of energy-boosting iron, black beans are a major power source. And with 15 grams of protein in one cup, they're a great way to replace meat on your menu. Aim for three 1-cup servings of dried beans per week. Canned beans have about the same nutritional value as dried, but may contain extra salt. Look for low-sodium varieties and rinse before using. Serve hot with brown rice or add to soups, salads and Tex-Mex dishes like chili.

Want to recharge your sex life?

In addition to these 7 power foods, Brock, author of *Dr. Ro's Ten Secrets to Livin' Healthy* (Bantam) prescribes an occasional treat of one to two ounces of dark chocolate, which in addition to being rich in antioxidants, contain a hormone compound that increases feel-good endorphins in the brain.

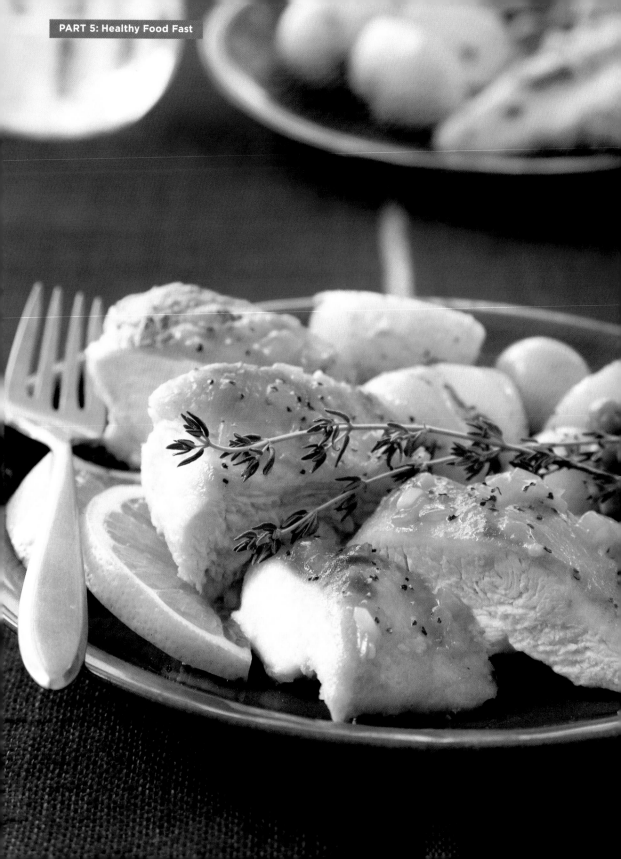

21 Delicious Meals

We've solved your evening what's-for-dinner dilemma with three weeks' worth of mouthwatering meals for the whole family: superfast salads, savory soups, hearty sandwiches, even meals special enough for company. Shop in advance, slow-cook on weekends, and make twice what you need to have heat-and-eat dishes prepped and ready. These easy, nutritious meals can fit any schedule—most can be pulled together in 20 minutes or less. Just take your pick. »

1 } Chicken With Lemon–Pepper Sauce

Makes 4 servings. ✳ Per serving: 242 calories, 10 grams fat, 86 milligrams cholesterol, 131 milligrams sodium, 8 grams carbohydrate, 30 grams protein.

4 boneless chicken breast halves

1 teaspoon salt, or to taste (optional)

1/2 teaspoon ground black pepper

1/4 cup all-purpose flour

1 tablespoon olive oil

1 tablespoon butter

1 shallot, minced

1/2 cup chicken broth

2 tablespoons lemon juice

1 teaspoon coarsely ground black pepper

Trim any visible fat from chicken. Sprinkle both sides with salt and pepper. On a plate or waxed paper, spread the flour. Coat chicken on both sides with flour, gently pressing to keep each piece intact. Lightly shake off any excess flour. Heat oil and butter in a large, heavy nonstick or well-seasoned skillet over medium heat. Add chicken with the tenderloin side in skillet; sauté 5 minutes (keeping fat hot but not burning). Using tongs, turn chicken; cook until firm to the touch and juices run clear, about another 5 minutes. Remove chicken from skillet; pour off all fat. Into skillet, stir shallot, chicken broth, lemon juice and coarse-ground pepper, scraping up browned bits. Over high heat, reduce mixture by half, about 2 minutes. Pour sauce over chicken. Delicious served with minted green peas and steamed new potatoes.

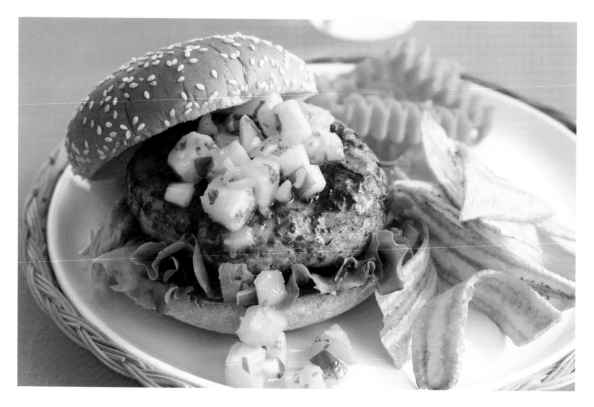

2} Jerk Turkey Burgers With Tropical Salsa

Makes 4 servings. ✳ Per serving: 329 calories, 11 grams fat, 90 milligrams cholesterol, 511 milligrams sodium, 32 grams carbohydrate, 24 grams protein.

TROPICAL SALSA:

$^3/_4$ cup diced fresh pineapple

$^3/_4$ cup diced fresh papaya

$^1/_2$ cup chopped red onion

1 tablespoon chopped cilantro

1 tablespoon lime juice

BURGERS:

4 ready-to-cook turkey burgers

2 tablespoons wet jerk seasoning or jerk sauce

Lettuce leaves

4 sandwich buns

To prepare Tropical Salsa: In bowl, mix all salsa ingredients. Cover and set aside for flavors to meld. Refrigerate if not used within an hour. Prepare and heat grill or grill pan. Season burgers with salt, if desired; brush with jerk seasoning. Grill until browned and no longer pink inside when tested with tip of knife, about 9 minutes, turning once. Toast buns, cut sides down, during last minutes of burger cooking time. Line bottom halves of buns with lettuce; top with patties. Spoon each with salsa; cover with top half of roll. Delicious with plantain chips and ginger beer.

3 } Creole Chicken + Herbed Rice

Makes 4 servings. ✳ Per serving: 282 calories, 10 grams fat, 63 milligrams cholesterol, 368 milligrams sodium, 23 grams carbohydrate, 26 grams protein.

CREOLE CHICKEN:

2 tablespoons olive oil

1 pound thin-sliced chicken cutlets

1/2 teaspoon salt (optional)

1/2 teaspoon ground black pepper

1/4 cup flour for dusting chicken

1 green bell pepper, sliced thin

1 onion, sliced thin

2 teaspoons minced garlic

14-ounce can stewed or Creole-seasoned tomatoes

HERBED RICE:

2 cups cooked rice

2 tablespoons chopped fresh parsley

1/2 teaspoon dried thyme

1/4 teaspoon salt (optional)

1 teaspoon olive oil

In medium-size skillet, heat oil over medium-high heat. Season chicken with salt and pepper; dredge in flour. Add to hot pan; let brown about 2 minutes on underside. Turn chicken cutlets; add bell pepper, onion and garlic to pan. Cover and cook 2 minutes. Remove chicken. Stir tomatoes into skillet. Return chicken to pan; cover and simmer 6 minutes. Adjust seasonings. Delicious served with herbed rice and baby carrots. To make Herbed Rice: In microwave-safe dish, mix 2 cups cooked rice, 2 tablespoons chopped fresh parsley, 1/2 teaspoon dried thyme, 1/4 teaspoon salt (optional) and 1 teaspoon olive oil. Heat on high about 3 minutes.

4 } Quick Chicken Soup

Makes 4 servings. ✳ Per serving: 341 calories, 10 grams fat, 64 milligrams cholesterol, 628 milligrams sodium, 34 grams carbohydrate, 29 grams protein.

1 tablespoon oil

1 cup chopped onion

1/2 cup chopped celery

2 teaspoons minced garlic

3/4 pound cooked chicken, torn into shreds or cubed

2 medium-size carrots, sliced thin

1 quart (4 cups) low-fat chicken broth

1 dried bay leaf

1/2 teaspoon salt (optional)

1/2 teaspoon ground black pepper

1 tablespoon chopped fresh parsley or 1 teaspoon parsley flakes

1 cup fusilli (corkscrew) pasta or other medium-size shape (about 4 ounces)

1 cup frozen green peas, thawed

In Dutch oven, heat oil; sauté onion, celery and garlic, about 1 minute. Add chicken, carrots, broth, salt, pepper, parsley and bay leaf. Over high heat, bring to boil. Stir in pasta and peas. When liquid returns to boil, reduce heat to simmer. Cook uncovered, stirring occasionally to prevent sticking, until pasta is done and vegetables are tender, about 8 to 10 minutes (depending on pasta type). Discard bay leaf.

Grilled Smoked Turkey Sandwiches

Makes 4 servings. ✳ *Per serving: 372 calories, 9 grams fat, 75 milligrams cholesterol, 647 milligrams sodium, 35 grams carbohydrate, 38 grams protein.*

8 slices sandwich bread

4 tablespoons honey Dijon mustard

½ pound sliced low-fat Swiss-style cheese, or Gruyére or Muenster

½ pound sliced low-sodium smoked or roasted turkey

12 arugula leaves

1 tablespoon butter or oil

Place 4 bread slices on work surface; spread each with 1 tablespoon mustard. Beginning and ending with cheese, equally divide the cheese, turkey and arugula leaves over each bread slice. Top with remaining bread. Heat large skillet, grill pan, griddle or sandwich press (panini). Grease surface with butter or oil. Cook sandwiches until bread is nicely browned on each side and cheese is melted, about 3 to 4 minutes each side, in uncovered pan. Cut sandwiches in half. Delicious with tomato soup.

Corn + Shrimp Soup

Makes 4 servings. ✳ *Per serving: 287 calories, 8 grams fat, 180 milligrams cholesterol, 342 milligrams sodium, 26 grams carbohydrate, 29 grams protein.*

1 tablespoon olive oil

1 cup chopped onion

1 rib celery, diced

2 cups fresh corn kernels or 10-ounce package frozen corn

1 tablespoon flour

8-ounce bottle clam juice

1 cup water

1 dried bay leaf

1 pound raw peeled, deveined shrimp

1 cup milk or half-and-half

1 teaspoon salt, or to taste (optional)

½ teaspoon ground black pepper, or to taste

1 tablespoon chopped fresh chives

In large saucepan, heat olive oil. Add onion, celery and corn; cook 5 minutes. Sprinkle flour over mixture; cook for 1 minute. Stir in clam juice, water and bay leaf; bring to boil. Add shrimp; cook until done, about 3 minutes. Stir in milk; season with salt and pepper. Heat briefly. Ladle into bowls or tureen; garnish with chives and serve immediately.

Eat Healthy Tip Choose foods that are the least processed (fresh vegetables, legumes, natural seasonings and whole grains) to be at the heart of your diet. They retain more of their nutritional value. Trying new recipes helps you learn more ways to prepare them.

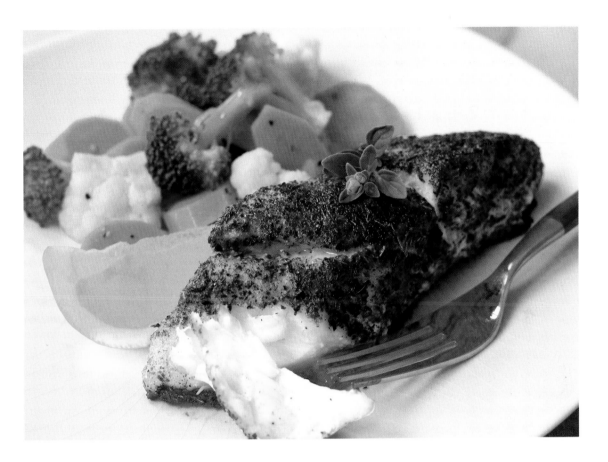

7 } Pepper-Crusted Grouper With Vegetable Medley

Makes 4 servings. ✳ *Per serving: 236 calories, 9 grams fat, 42 milligrams cholesterol, 103 milligrams sodium, 16 grams carbohydrate, 26 grams protein.*

1 pound grouper fillets

1 teaspoon salt (optional)

3 to 4 tablespoons pepper rub or seasoning blend

1 tablespoon dried oregano, rosemary or other herb

2 tablespoons olive oil, divided

12-ounce package frozen mixed vegetables

Optional garnishes: oregano sprig, lemon wedges

Sprinkle fish with salt. Spread rub and dried herb on a plate. Gently press fish into pepper mixture to adhere to rub; turn over and repeat to completely coat. Heat large nonstick skillet over medium heat. Add half (1 tablespoon) of the oil and swirl it to coat pan. When pan is hot, lightly shake any loose coating from fish; place fish in pan. Cook until bottom side is crusty, about 3 minutes (for fish about ½ inch thick). When turning fish to other side, add remaining oil. Cook until crusty. As fish cooks, microwave vegetables. Serve fish with or atop vegetables. Garnish with herb and lemon wedges.

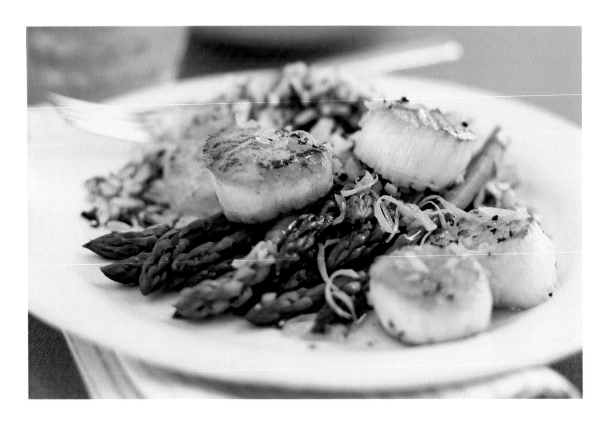

8} Seared Scallops in Lemon–Butter Sauce With Asparagus

Makes 4 servings. ✳ *Per serving: 184 calories, 9 grams fat, 52 milligrams cholesterol, 190 milligrams sodium, 6 grams carbohydrate, 20 grams protein.*

1 bunch asparagus, cleaned, stem ends trimmed

2 teaspoons olive oil

1 pound sea scallops

½ teaspoon salt (optional)

¼ teaspoon ground black or red pepper

1 tablespoon chopped shallot (available freeze-dried in spice section)

2 tablespoons butter

2 tablespoons lemon juice (juice of one lemon)

In medium-size skillet, bring 1 cup salted water to boil. Add asparagus, laying flat; cook until crisp-tender, about 6 minutes for medium-size spears. Meanwhile, heat olive oil in large nonstick skillet. Pat scallops dry. Season with salt and pepper. Cook 3 minutes per side over medium-high heat; remove and keep warm. Add shallot to skillet; cook 30 seconds. Stir in butter; cook until lightly browned, about 2 minutes. Turn off heat; add lemon juice, taking care to avoid splattering. Drain asparagus well; arrange on plates. Place scallops on top of asparagus. Drizzle with butter sauce. For an optional garnish, sprinkle with lemon zest (shredded peel).

9} Broiled Lamb Chops + Spring Vegetables

Makes 4 servings. ✳ *Per serving: 371 calories, 21 grams fat, 109 milligrams cholesterol, 286 milligrams sodium, 13 grams carbohydrate, 33 grams protein.*

1 cup whole fresh baby carrots

1 $1/2$ cups fresh or frozen green peas, thawed

$1/2$ teaspoon dried thyme or 2 teaspoons fresh

8 lamb chops, each with only 2 ounces edible
   meat (4 ounces per serving)

1 teaspoon salt (optional)

$1/4$ teaspoon ground black pepper

2 tablespoons grainy Dijon mustard

Optional garnish: mint leaves (chopped or whole)

To small saucepan, add baby carrots and $3/4$ cup water; bring to boil. Cook 5 minutes. Add peas and thyme; simmer 5 minutes. Meanwhile, heat broiler. Trim all visible fat from lamb chops. Season chops with salt and pepper; brush each side with mustard. Place on broiler pan 3 to 4 inches from heat. Cook 3 to 4 minutes per side, turning once, for medium doneness. Sprinkle vegetables with mint. Delicious served with steamed small red-skinned potatoes.

10} Linguine With White Clam Sauce

Makes 4 servings. ✳ *Per serving: 339 calories, 8 grams fat, 40 milligrams cholesterol, 454 milligrams sodium, 47 grams carbohydrate, 20 grams protein.*

$1/2$ pound linguine

1 tablespoon olive oil

2 teaspoons minced garlic

3 tablespoons chopped fresh parsley

8-ounce bottle clam juice

2 tablespoons lemon juice

12 littleneck clams, scrubbed, rinsed in several
   changes of water

10-ounce can minced clams with liquid

1 tablespoon butter

Garnishes: red-pepper flakes, grated
   Parmesan cheese

Cook linguine according to package directions. In large pot, heat oil; cook garlic until golden, 1 minute. Add 2 tablespoons chopped parsley, clam juice and lemon juice. Simmer 3 minutes. Add littleneck clams and cover. Cook until clams open, about 3 minutes; discard any unopened ones. Add canned clams; bring to boil. Stir in butter. Drain linguine; add to pot, mixing well, or place drained pasta in bowl and top with sauce. Sprinkle with remaining parsley and garnishes.

Quick Tip:
To bring water
to a faster boil,
put a lid on it.

11 } Rigatoni With Sausage + Peppers

Makes 4 servings. ✳ *Per serving: 505 calories, 9 grams fat, 12 milligrams cholesterol, 1,003 milligrams sodium, 88 grams carbohydrate, 19 grams protein.*

12 ounces tube pasta such as rigatoni, penne or ziti

1 tablespoon olive oil

½ pound precooked, low-fat smoked sausage, cut into ½-inch-thick slices

1 cup chopped green bell pepper

1 cup chopped onion

16-ounce jar marinara sauce

Optional garnishes: chopped flat-leaf parsley, grated Parmesan cheese

Cook pasta according to package directions. Meanwhile, in large skillet, heat oil. Add sausage, peppers and onion. Cook 5 minutes, stirring occasionally until peppers and onion are tender and the sausage is heated through. Add sauce; bring to simmer. Stir in the drained pasta. If desired, sprinkle with parsley; pass cheese at table. Delicious served with a crisp green salad.

12 } Grilled Salmon With Mango–Peach Salsa

Makes 4 servings. ✳ *Per serving: 253 calories, 16 grams fat, 67 milligrams cholesterol, 262 milligrams sodium, 4 grams carbohydrate, 23 grams protein.*

Juice of 2 limes (about 4 tablespoons)

3 tablespoons finely chopped fresh cilantro

1 tablespoon olive oil

1 pound salmon fillet, cut into 4 serving portions

1 teaspoon sea salt (optional)

Freshly cracked or ground black pepper

1 tablespoon garlic flakes or 1 teaspoon garlic powder

½ cup prepared mango–peach salsa

In large zip-type food storage bag, mix ½ of lime juice, ¼ of cilantro and olive oil. Add salmon; turn bag to coat fish. If desired, marinate 30 minutes or up to 8 hours in refrigerator. Meanwhile, to enhance salsa, add remaining juice and cilantro. Chill, if desired. To cook salmon: Heat countertop grill or grill pan. Remove salmon from bag; season with salt, pepper and garlic. In covered grill, cook 7 to 9 minutes. In grill pan, cook about 5 minutes per side. To sear, transfer fillets to broilerproof pan; broil 1 to 3 minutes, watching closely. Plate salmon; top with salsa. Serve with mixture of steamed asparagus, sliced avocado and strips of yellow bell pepper.

Add Waves of Flavor With seasonings, aim to enhance, not overwhelm, the subtle flavors of fish. Citrus fruits—lemon, lime, orange— are classic accents. As for herbs, dill, rosemary, fennel and marjoram go well with fish. For zip, add garlic, ginger, soy sauce or bottled vinaigrette.

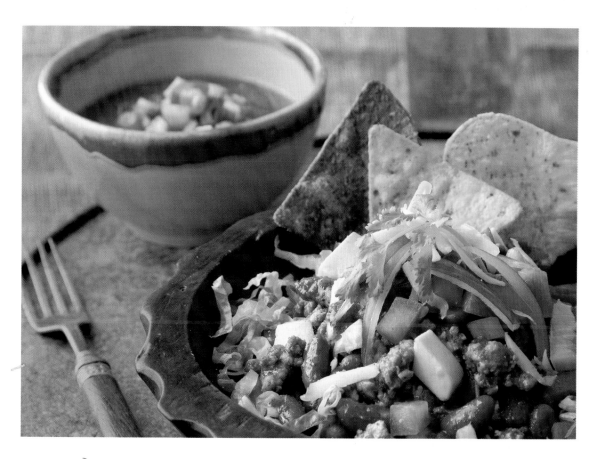

13} Tex-Mex Taco Salad

*Makes 4 servings. * Per serving: 309 calories, 13 grams fat, 70 milligrams cholesterol, 305 milligrams sodium, 24 grams carbohydrate, 25 grams protein.*

1 tablespoon canola oil

½ to 1 cup chopped onion

2 teaspoons chopped garlic

³⁄₄ pound lean ground turkey or beef

14-ounce can no-salt-added stewed tomatoes

15-ounce can kidney beans, drained, rinsed

1 tablespoon chili powder

1 teaspoon ground cumin

½ teaspoon salt, or to taste

½ teaspoon cayenne pepper or hot pepper sauce

2 tablespons chopped cilantro

4 cups shredded lettuce

½ cup reduced-fat shredded Mexican-style cheese

Optional toppings: sliced or cubed avocado, tomato, red onion, scallions, tortilla chips (try different flavors), salsa

Heat oil in nonstick skillet over medium heat. Add onion and garlic; sauté about 1 minute. Add ground meat; brown, stirring, until cooked through, about 5 minutes. Pour off pan drippings. Stir in tomatoes with liquid, beans, chili powder, cumin, salt and pepper. Cook, stirring several times until heated through, about 3 minutes. Add cilantro. Serve meat mixture atop lettuce. Sprinkle with cheese and optional toppings of choice.

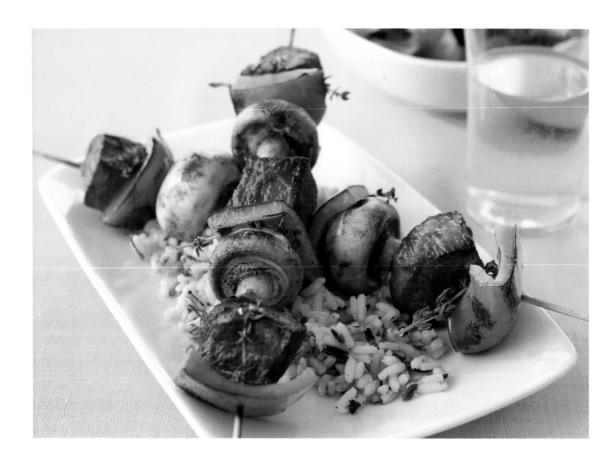

14 } Spicy Kebobs With Wild Rice

Makes 4 serving. ✶ *Per serving: 276 calories, 7 grams fat, 46 milligrams cholesterol, 365 milligrams sodium, 22 grams carbohydrate, 28 grams protein.*

8-ounce pouch long-grain and wild-rice blend (cooks in 90 seconds)

¼ cup low-fat Italian salad dressing

1 tablespoon Tabasco Chipotle Pepper Sauce

1 pound top loin, sirloin or top round beef, cut into cubes

1 bell pepper, cut into 1-inch pieces

8 mushrooms

1 onion, cut into 8 wedges

Thyme or other fresh herb sprigs (optional)

8 metal or wooden skewers

1 teaspoon salt (optional)

Cook rice according to package directions. Prepare and heat grill or grill pan. In large bowl or large food storage bag, combine salad dressing and hot sauce. Add beef, vegetables and herbs; mix well. Assemble on skewers, alternating beef and vegetables; add twists of herb sprigs. Sprinkle salt over kebobs. Place them on grill; for medium doneness, cook about 10 minutes, turning once. Serve over wild-rice blend.

15 } Ginger Beef + Vegetable Stir-Fry

Makes 4 servings. ✻ *Per serving: 370 calories, 12 grams fat, 36 milligrams cholesterol, 338 milligrams sodium, 44 grams carbohydrate, 22 grams protein.*

1 cup instant brown rice

1 tablespoon vegetable oil

2 scallions, sliced thin

2 teaspoons minced garlic

1 tablespoon grated fresh ginger

1 teaspoon salt (optional)

1 teaspoon cornstarch

$3/4$ pound stir-fry beef

1 red bell pepper, sliced

3 cups broccoli florets

2 cups sliced mushrooms

2 tablespoons low-sodium soy sauce

$1/2$ cup low-sodium low-fat beef broth or water

Prepare rice according to package directions. In large nonstick skillet, heat oil over medium-high heat. Add scallions, garlic and ginger; cook 1 minute. Sprinkle salt and cornstarch on beef; add to skillet. Cook until browned, about 3 minutes; remove meat from pan. Add vegetables to skillet; stir-fry 1 minute. Add soy sauce and beef broth. Cover; simmer 3 minutes. Stir in cooked beef. Serve over rice or noodles.

16 } Peppercorn Steak With Salad + Cheese Croutons

Makes 4 servings. ✻ *Per crouton: 113 calories, 4 grams fat, 15 milligrams cholesterol, 240 milligrams sodium, 15 grams carbohydrate, 3 grams protein.* ✻ *Per serving, steak only: 178 calories, 9 grams fat, 50 milligrams cholesterol, 280 milligrams sodium, 1 gram carbohydrate, 23 grams protein.*

STEAK:

1 pound beef skirt steak

$1/4$ to $1/2$ teaspoon salt

1 tablespoon cracked black
  pepper

CHEESE CROUTONS:

Baguette of French bread

Boursin cheese

Season steak with salt. Press pepper into both sides of steak. Place steak on rack in broiler pan so surface of meat is 2 to 3 inches from heat. Broil 10 minutes for medium doneness, turning once. Delicious served with tossed salad and Cheese Croutons. Cut baguette of French bread into 12 slices. Top each with about a teaspoon of Boursin cheese. Toast briefly under broiler.

Steak Done Right

Bright red in the middle or browned right through? Use this guide for broiled or grilled 1-inch-thick steaks over medium heat:

Rare: about 3 to 4 minutes per side (135°F–140°F)

Medium-rare: about 4 to 5 minutes per side (145°F)

Medium: about 5 to 6 minutes per side (160°F)

Well-done: about 7 to 8 minutes per side (170°F)

17 } Goat Cheese + Bell Pepper Pizza

Makes 4 servings. ✳ *Per serving: 330 calories, 14 grams fat, 10 milligrams cholesterol, 638 milligrams sodium, 43 grams carbohydrate, 14 grams protein.*

Packaged presliced mixed bell peppers

1 cup sliced mushrooms

1/2 cup diced red onion

1 tablespoon oil

8 ounces low-fat soft goat cheese

1 teaspoon minced garlic

1 teaspoon chopped fresh oregano leaves

Freshly ground black pepper

12-inch prebaked pizza shell

Heat oven to 450°F. In nonstick skillet, sauté bell peppers, mushrooms and onion in oil about 4 minutes. Meanwhile, in bowl, mix cheese, garlic, oregano and black pepper. Spread crust with about 3/4 of the crumbled cheese mixture. Top with sautéed vegetables and remaining cheese. Bake until crust is crisp and cheese softens, about 8 minutes.

---

18 } Smoky Two Bean Chili

Makes 5 servings. ✳ *Per serving: 236 calories, 8 grams fat, 0 milligrams cholesterol, 562 milligrams sodium, 36 grams carbohydrate, 10 grams protein.*

2 tablespoons olive oil

1 cup chopped onion

2 cups chopped bell peppers

1 cup sliced baby carrots

2 teaspoons minced garlic

14-to-16-ounce can garbanzo beans, rinsed, drained

14-to-16-ounce can red kidney beans, rinsed, drained

2 chipotle peppers, chopped

16-ounce can whole tomatoes, undrained, chopped

8-ounce can tomato sauce

2 tablespoons chili powder

1 teaspoon ground cumin

1/2 to 1 cup water (depending on desired consistency)

In 4-quart Dutch oven, heat oil. Sauté onion, bell peppers, carrots and garlic, about 3 minutes. Stir in remaining ingredients. Cover and simmer 8 minutes. Great served with warm corn tortillas.

Meatless Mondays If the hardest part of eating better—more fresh foods and less saturated fat—is getting started, here's a boost: Kick off the week by going meatless each Monday. Build your main meal around vegetables, fruits, whole grains and occasional seafood. This way you won't feel you're giving up a thing.

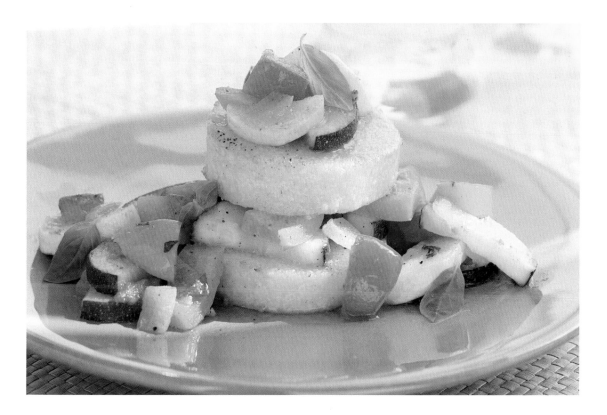

19 } Polenta + Summer Vegetables

Makes 4 servings. ✳ *Per serving: 142 calories, 3 grams fat, 0 milligrams*
cholesterol, 361 milligrams sodium, 26 grams carbohydrate, 4 grams protein.

2 teaspoons oil

1 small onion, chopped

1 medium-size zucchini, halved lengthwise,
  sliced crosswise

1 medium-size yellow summer squash, halved
  lengthwise, sliced crosswise

1 small orange bell pepper, seeded, cut into chunks

1 to 2 medium-size ripe tomatoes, chopped

1 teaspoon salt (optional)

$^{1}/_{2}$ teaspoon ground black pepper

2 tablespoons chopped fresh basil (and whole
  leaves for garnish)

1-pound tube-package precooked polenta,
  drained, sliced

Olive oil cooking spray

In large saucepan, heat oil; sauté onion until wilted, about 1 minute. Stir in remaining vegetables. Over
medium-low heat, cover and cook in released juices, about 5 minutes. Add salt, pepper and chopped basil. Coat
polenta slices lightly with cooking spray. In large nonstick skillet, cook polenta until lightly browned, about 3
minutes per side. To serve: Place a polenta slice, top with mixed vegetables, another slice of polenta and veggies.

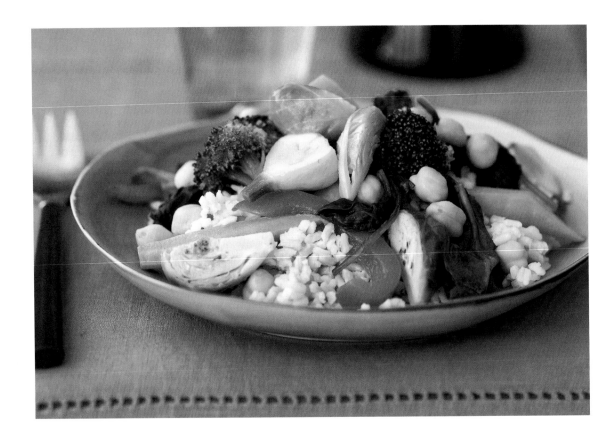

20 } Brown Rice + Sautéed Vegetables

Makes 4 servings. ✳ *Per serving: 303 calories, 6 grams fat, 0 milligrams cholesterol,*
308 milligrams sodium, 55 grams carbohydrate, 9 grams protein.

1 cup uncooked brown rice

2 cups water

1/4 teaspoon salt (optional)

1 tablespoon vegetable oil

1 cup sliced carrots

1 cup broccoli florets

1 cup sliced zucchini

1 red bell pepper, seeded, cut into strips or chunks

1 cup drained chickpeas (garbanzo beans)

1/2 cup chicken or vegetable broth

2 cups baby spinach leaves

In heavy-bottomed saucepan, combine rice, water and salt. Over medium-high heat, bring to boil. Reduce heat to low; cover and cook until liquid is absorbed, about 45 minutes. In large nonstick skillet, heat oil over medium-high heat. Add carrots, broccoli, zucchini, pepper and chickpeas, stirring occasionally; cook until crisp-tender, about 5 minutes. Add broth and spinach; cook until spinach is wilted and heated through, about 2 minutes. Serve over rice.

21} Barbecued Tofu And Soba Noodles

Makes 4 servings. ✱ Per serving: 389 calories, 14 grams fat, 0 cholesterol, 421 milligrams sodium, 52 grams carbohydrate, 23 grams protein.

8 ounces soba, udon or noodles of choice

14-ounce package extra-firm tofu

1/4 cup barbecue sauce

2 tablespoons canola oil

2 chopped scallions

8 ounces sliced mushrooms

1 cup fresh spinach

2 teaspoons light soy sauce

Optional garnish: trimmed or chopped scallions

Cook noodles according to package directions. Meanwhile, cut tofu crosswise into inch-wide slices, then lay flat and cut each into 2 or 3 pieces. Place in shallow dish; coat with 2 tablespoons barbecue sauce; set aside. In large nonstick skillet, heat 1 tablespoon oil until hot. Cook scallions and mushrooms about 2 minutes. Add spinach and soy sauce; cook until spinach wilts, about 2 minutes. Remove from pan to bowl; keep warm. Wipe skillet; heat remaining oil. Cook tofu until golden brown, 2 minutes per side. Toss with remaining barbecue sauce. Drain noodles; transfer to platter or plates. Top with mushroom mixture, tofu and garnish.

Time-saving Cooking Tips

Reach for ready-made. To pull together kebobs even faster than the recipe we featured, check supermarket meat departments and butcher shops for the ready-to-cook kind.

Cook food in an instant. Getting the best nutrients in your food doesn't necessarily mean opting for slow cooking. For example, if you haven't heard the nutritional buzz, brown is the new white—especially for rice. Brown rice offers three times the fiber of white, and a megadose of vitamins and minerals. But regular brown rice requires a longer cooking time, about 45 minutes, so when you're in a rush, consider quick-cooking or instant versions. They can be ready 90 seconds.

Slaw down the process. Packaged coleslaw—a mix of washed, shredded, ready-to-eat green cabbage, carrots and sometimes red cabbage—offers multiple shortcuts and is delicious year-round. Toss in seasonal fruit, like pears, apples, pineapple, peaches, even raisins. Or add extras like chopped broccoli or cauliflower, cherry tomatoes and nuts. To get even more out of the bag: Cook the cabbage mix in a quick stir-fry, soup or side dish.

Start Strong, Finish Sweet

4 Great Ways to Begin Your Day

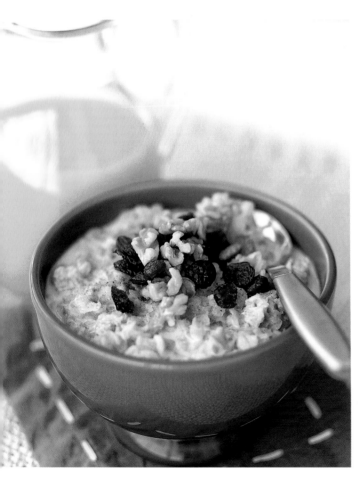

1. Oatmeal With Dried Cherries + Walnuts

Makes 4 servings. ✳ *Per serving: 184 calories, 7 grams fat, 0 milligrams cholesterol, 1 milligram sodium, 28 grams carbohydrate, 6 grams protein. For best results, follow the package directions for cooking oatmeal or use this technique. For creamier texture and taste, cook cereal in milk or a mixture of milk and water.*

1 1/2 cups old-fashioned oats

3 cups water, skim milk or a combination

1/4 teaspoon salt (optional)

1/2 teaspoon ground cinnamon

1/4 cup dried cherries or raisins

1/4 cup coarsely chopped walnuts

In heavy saucepan, combine oats, water and (if desired) salt; mix well. Over medium-high heat, bring to boil. Reduce heat to low; cook until tender and no taste of raw starch remains, about 15 minutes. Spoon into bowls. Sprinkle with cinnamon, cherries and walnuts. Serve with sugar and milk or cream, if desired.

2. Cheese + Spinach Egg White Omelet

*Makes 4 servings * Per serving: 113 calories, 4 grams fat, 10 milligrams cholesterol, 906 milligrams sodium, 4 grams carbohydrate, 15 grams protein.*

10-ounce package frozen
    chopped spinach
4 tablespoons light
    cream cheese
1 teaspoon salt, divided (optional)
1/2 teaspoon ground black
    pepper or cayenne pepper
12 large egg whites or 8 ounces
    liquid egg whites
Cooking spray
2 tablespoons grated
    Parmesan cheese

Cook spinach as directed on package; drain well. In a large bowl, combine spinach, cream cheese and half of the salt and pepper, then set aside. In another large bowl, whisk egg whites with remaining salt and pepper. Coat nonstick skillet with cooking spray; heat. Add 1/4 egg mixture. Cook until edges begin to set, about 1 minute. Occasionally lift cooked egg around edge to allow raw egg to flow underneath. Cook until set, though moist on top, about 2 minutes. Add spinach mixture; sprinkle with cheese. Cover and cook until top is done, about 1 minute. Fold in half.

3. Breakfast Parfait

*Makes 2 servings. * Per serving: 380 calories, 17 grams fat, 7 milligrams cholesterol, 102 milligrams sodium, 47 grams carbohydrate, 12 grams protein.*

1/2 cup no-sugar-added granola
1 cup of your favorite low-fat yogurt
1 banana, peeled, sliced
1 tablespoon honey
1/4 cup orange juice

In a bowl or parfait glass, alternate granola, yogurt and banana slices. Drizzle with honey and orange juice.

4. Mango Madness Smoothie

*Make 2 servings. * Per serving: 223 calories, 2 grams of fat, 4 milligrams cholesterol, 76 milligrams sodium, 50 grams carbohydrate, 6 grams protein.*

1/2 cup skim or soy milk
1/2 cup low-fat mango-flavored yogurt
2 1/2 cups frozen diced fresh mango
    (To freeze mango: Peel, then slice
    fruit away from long seed; dice. Place
    in plastic bag and freeze until firm.)
1 tablespoon fresh lime juice
1 teaspoon grated fresh ginger
Several ice cubes

In blender container, combine milk and yogurt. Add frozen diced mango, lime juice and ginger. With blender running, add ice cubes one at a time until incorporated and of desired consistency. Pour into glasses and serve immediately.

4 Guilt-Free Dessert Delights

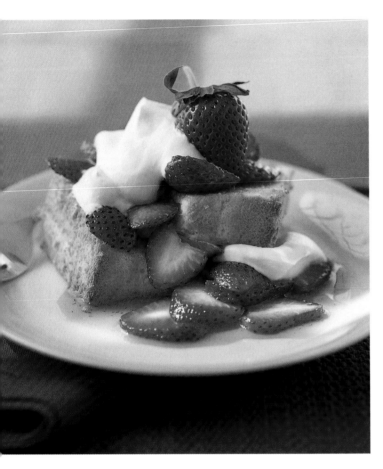

1 quart ripe strawberries,
  rinsed
1/4 cup granulated sugar
1/2 cup heavy cream, chilled
2 teaspoons pure vanilla extract
2 tablespoons confectioner's sugar
  or extra-fine sugar
15-ounce ready-made angel
  food cake, cut into 16 slices

Set aside eight whole strawberries for garnish. With tip of a huller or paring knife, remove the hulls from remaining berries. Cut berries into slices. Place strawberries in medium-size bowl; sprinkle with granulated sugar. Cover and let stand at room temperature until sweetened and juicy, at least 30 minutes. To whip cream: Chill large bowl and electric-mixer beaters or manual beater in freezer for about 30 minutes. On medium speed, whip cream in chilled bowl until soft peaks form, about 2 to 4 minutes. Add vanilla and sprinkle with confectioner's sugar. Increase mixer speed to high; whip until stiff peaks take shape, another 2 to 3 minutes. To assemble: Place first cake slice on each plate. Top cake with sliced berries, juice and whipped cream. Cover with another slice of cake and berries. Top with a dollop of whipped cream; garnish with a whole strawberry.

1. The Best Summer Fruit Shortcake

This no-bake version of the classic dessert is light as a cloud. It's simply made with store-bought angel food cake, your choice of ripe berries or sliced fruit, and real whipped cream ✳ Makes 8 servings. Per serving: 246 calories, 6 grams fat, 20 milligrams cholesterol, 405 milligrams sodium, 45 grams carbohydrate, 4 grams protein.

2. Melon Grantias

Makes about 12 servings ✳ Per serving: 64 calories, 1 gram fat, 0 milligrams cholesterol, 1 milligram sodium, 16 grams carbohydrate, 1 gram protein. ✳ For layered parfaits, divide recipe in half or thirds and use different melons.

1 cup water
1/4 to 1 cup sugar, according to taste
4 cups peeled, seeded ripe melon,
    cut into large chunks
1 tablespoon lemon juice

In small saucepan, heat water and sugar until sugar dissolves; let cool. In food processor, combine melon, lemon juice and sugar syrup. Puree until smooth. Pour mixture into baking pan. Freeze 1 to 2 hours, stirring every half hour until frozen solid. Break into chunks; return to food processor. Process mixture until smooth. Return to baking pan and freeze 20 to 30 minutes. To serve: Scrape and spoon into chilled parfait glasses or bowls.

3. Pears Poached in Wine With Orange Zest

Makes 4 servings ✳ Per serving: 185 calories, 1 gram fat, 0 milligrams cholesterol, 6 milligrams sodium, 28 grams carbohydrate, 1 gram protein.

4 firm, ripe pears with stems
2 cups sweet white wine (a sauterne
    works well)

1/4 cup orange juice
1 cinnamon stick
Long peel from navel orange, cut into thin strips
Optional garnish: mint leaves

Using small end of melon baller or paring knife, cut cores from bottom ends of pears, leaving stems intact. Peel pears. In Dutch oven or large saucepan, stand pears with space between them. Pour wine and orange juice over pears. Bring poaching liquid to boil; reduce heat to medium-low. Cover pan and gently simmer pears, basting occasionally with liquid, until tender, about 25 minutes. Remove pan from heat. If time permits, allow pears to cool in juice, spooning occasionally. Using slotted spoon, transfer them to stand in center of 4 dessert plates. To make sauce: Add cinnamon stick and orange zest to liquid in pot. Bring mixture to boil; lower heat and simmer until sauce is reduced. Spoon sauce over pears; garnish each with orange zest and mint leaves, if desired.

4. Juicy Baked Apples

Makes 4 servings. ✳ Per apple: 327 calories, 5 grams fat, 0 milligrams cholesterol, 15 milligrams sodium, 73 grams carbohydrate, 3 grams protein.

4 large cooking apples, such as Cortland or Rome
1 cup dried-fruit and nut granola
1/2 cup maple syrup or maple-flavored syrup,
    or 1 cup apple juice

Heat oven to 350°F. Remove apple cores without cutting all the way through to the bottom. Beginning at top, peel each 1/4 way down. Stand apples in shallow 9-inch baking dish. Spoon 1/4 cup granola into cavity of each apple. Pour maple syrup over and around apples. Bake apples, basting occasionally with syrup in dish, until very tender, about 50 minutes. Serve warm or cover and refrigerate to serve chilled. Delicious served with frozen vanilla yogurt.

Just Like Home

Spicy Shrimp With Grits

Makes 4 servings ∗ Per serving: 322 calories, 13 grams fat, 145 milligrams cholesterol, 435 milligrams sodium, 30 grams carbohydrate, 20 grams protein.

$3/4$ cup quick-cooking grits

$1/4$ cup chopped green onions

1 tablespoons olive oil

4 ounces precooked smoked sausage,
   sliced or diced

$1/2$ cup chopped onion

$1/2$ cup chopped mixed bell peppers

1 teaspoon minced garlic

$3/4$ pound large shrimp, peeled, deveined
   (tails intact, if desired)

2 plum tomatoes, chopped

$1/4$ teaspoon salt (optional)

$1/4$ teaspoon freshly ground black pepper

1 teaspoon Old Bay seasoning

Cook grits according to package directions. Stir in green onions; set aside. Meanwhile, in large skillet, heat oil. Add sausage, onion, bell peppers and garlic. Sauté about 3 minutes. Pour off fat. Add shrimp, tomatoes, salt, pepper and seasoning. Cover; cook until shrimp are pink and opaque, about 5 minutes. Spoon shrimp mixture over grits; serve immediately.

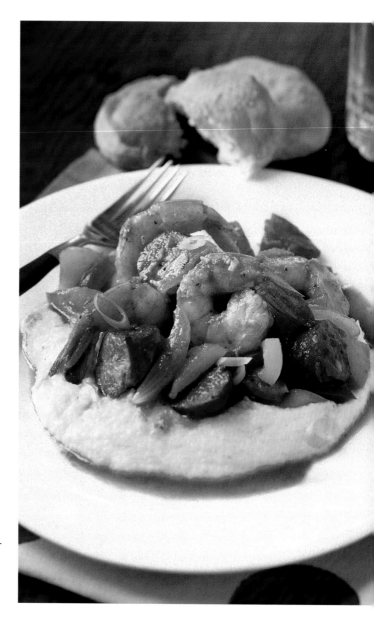

Cookin'

We improved the profile of family favorites by keeping fat and calories to minimum. Bet you can't tell what's missing. »

Black-Eyed Peas With Smoked Turkey

Makes 4 servings ✳ *Per main-dish serving (peas and turkey): 271 calories, 7 grams fat, 43 milligrams cholesterol, 770 milligrams sodium, 26 grams carbohydrate, 25 grams protein.*

1 tablespoon canola oil

1/2 cup sliced or chopped yellow onion

1/2 cup chopped green/red bell pepper

8-ounce piece ready-to-eat smoked turkey, diced (leg or thigh meat)

Two 15-ounce cans black-eyed peas, drained, rinsed

2 teaspoons fresh thyme leaves or 1/2 teaspoon dried

1/4 cup chicken broth or vegetable broth

In medium-size saucepan, heat oil; sauté onion, bell pepper and turkey until vegetables begin to soften, about 2 minutes. Stir in black-eyed peas, thyme and broth; simmer about 8 minutes. Delicious served with brown rice and collards. Note: Cook frozen collards according to package directions. Sprinkle with 2 teaspoons wine vinegar and red pepper flakes. Try instant brown rice; it's more nutritious than white.

Oven "Fried" Chicken

Makes 8 servings ✳ *Per serving: 292 calories, 8 grams fat, 66 milligrams cholesterol, 195 milligrams sodium, 22 grams carbohydrate, 31 grams protein.*

6 boneless, skinless chicken-breast halves (about 4 ounces each)

2 egg whites

1/4 cup skim milk

1/2 cup unbleached all-purpose flour

2 teaspoons dried thyme or other herbs

1 teaspoon salt (optional)

1/2 teaspoon ground black pepper

1 cup finely crushed cornflakes or dried bread crumbs

Nonstick cooking spray

Heat oven to 400°F. In small bowl, beat egg whites and milk. In large plastic food-storage bag, combine flour and seasonings; mix well. Add breast halves, 1 or 2 at a time, to flour mixture, then dredge in egg white mixture and crumbs until coated. Arrange in single layer on 15-by-10-inch baking pan or baking sheet. Spray chicken lightly with cooking spray. Bake 10 minutes; turn chicken and bake on other side until no longer pink in center, about 10 additional minutes.

Lighten Up...

Try these tips to bring out the best of traditional dishes: ✳ **Trim fat before cooking, pour off fat during cooking, and use a defatting cup to keep sauces trim.** ✳ **Use lean cuts of meat, and limit portions to 3 to 4 ounces.** ✳ **Bake, roast, broil or grill instead of deep-frying.** ✳ **To brown or sauté, use 2 tablespoons of healthy oils, such as olive, or spritz with cooking spray.** ✳ **Season greens and beans with smoked turkey instead of fatty meats, and use herbs or zest instead of salt.**

Baked Macaroni + Cheese

Makes 6 servings * *Per serving: 303 calories, 11 grams fat, 22 milligrams cholesterol, 316 milligrams sodium, 35 grams carbohydrate, 19 grams protein.*

2 cups uncooked macaroni

2 tablespoons tub margarine

2 tablespoons minced onion

1 tablespoon unbleached
  all-purpose flour

1/4 teaspoon dry mustard

1/8 teaspoon ground white pepper

2 cups skim milk

8 ounces shredded 50 percent
  reduced-fat cheddar cheese

1 ripe tomato, sliced thin

1 teaspoon dried or 1 tablespoon
  fresh parsley flakes

Cook macaroni according to label directions. Meanwhile, heat oven to 400°F. Melt margarine in saucepan over medium-high heat. Add onion, flour, dry mustard and white pepper. Slowly stir in milk. Cook, stirring frequently, until smooth and hot, about 8 minutes. Add cheese and stir about 10 seconds. When macaroni is tender, drain in colander; transfer to lightly greased or sprayed 2-quart casserole. Pour cheese sauce over macaroni and toss lightly to mix. Arrange tomato slices on top of macaroni. Sprinkle parsley over tomatoes. Bake, uncovered, 20 minutes.

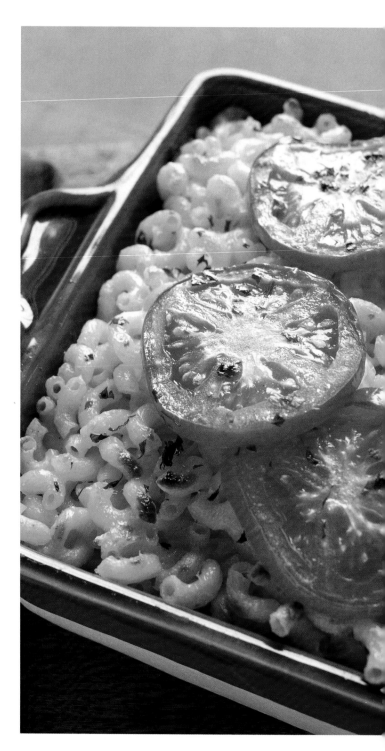

Light Potato Salad

Makes 12 servings ＊ *Per serving: 207 calories, 9 grams fat, 59 milligrams cholesterol, 209 milligrams sodium, 28 grams carbohydrate, 5 grams protein. Our version of this southern classic is a real crowd-pleaser. We've substituted plain yogurt for some of the mayonnaise and cut back on calories—but not taste.*

3 pounds medium-size all-purpose
   potatoes (about 9 potatoes)
2 teaspoons salt for cooking
   potatoes (optional)
1/2 cup mayonnaise
1/2 cup plain yogurt
1 tablespoon prepared mustard
1/2 cup sweet pickle relish
1 teaspoon salt (optional)
1/2 teaspoon ground black pepper
3 large eggs, hard-cooked, chopped
2 large celery ribs, sliced thin
1/4 cup grated onion
Paprika

Place whole, unpeeled potatoes in 4- quart saucepan; cover with cold water. Add 2 teaspoons salt. Bring to boil over high heat. Reduce heat to low; cover and simmer until potatoes are tender, about 25 to 30 minutes. Drain potatoes; cool slightly. Using paring knife, pull away skin to peel; remove eyes and any spots. Cut potatoes into 3/4-inch cubes. In large bowl, blend dressing ingredients: mayonnaise, yogurt, mustard, relish, salt and pepper. Add potatoes, chopped eggs, celery and onion. Gently stir with wooden spoon or rubber spatula to mix and coat. (If you like, stir in celery seeds, chopped bell pepper, sliced olives, fresh dill, capers or diced pimiento.) If not serving immediately, cover and refrigerate. Optional garnishes: sprinkle of paprika, celery leaves.

Turkey Meat Loaf

Makes 10 servings ＊ *Per serving: 198 calories, 10 grams fat, 115 milligrams cholesterol, 272 milligrams sodium, 8 grams carbohydrate, 18 grams protein.*

1 tablespoon vegetable oil
1 medium-size onion, chopped
1 rib celery, sliced thin
1 small bell pepper, seeded, diced
2 to 3 garlic cloves, chopped fine
2 pounds ground turkey
1 cup fresh bread crumbs or
   3/4 cup dry bread crumbs
2 large eggs
1 teaspoon salt (optional)
1 teaspoon ground black pepper
1 teaspoon dried sage
1/4 cup low-fat milk
1/2 cup ketchup

In medium-size nonstick skillet, heat oil; add onion, celery and bell pepper. Sauté just until softened, about 5 minutes; add garlic and cook 2 minutes more. Meanwhile, heat oven to 350°F. In large bowl, place turkey, bread

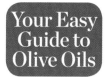

Your Easy Guide to Olive Oils

If you ever stare at the grocery shelf wondering what the difference is between types of olive oil, we break it down for you:

1. Extra Virgin Olive Oil offers the best of what olive oils are about. This first, chemical-free pressing is low in acid and the highest in flavor. It can be quite expensive. Use it for dressing salads and vegetable dishes, basting meats and seafood, and seasoning marinades and sauces. Instead of butter, dip or spread a bit of extra virgin on your bread.

2. Virgin Olive Oil is also a first-press oil but has higher ⟩⟩

crumbs and sautéed vegetables; set aside. In small bowl, using a whisk or fork, lightly beat eggs; mix in salt, black pepper, sage, milk and half of the ketchup until blended. Add egg mixture to turkey in large bowl. Using wooden spoon or hands, mix ingredients until uniform (do not over-mix). Turn mixture onto work surface. With wet hands, pat into an approximately 9-by-5-inch loaf shape. Place in foil-lined (for easy cleanup) shallow baking pan. Or lightly pack mixture into 9-by-5-inch loaf pan, slightly rounding top. Spread remaining ketchup over top. Bake about 50 minutes or until internal temperature reaches 170°F. Let stand 10 minutes before slicing.

Oven "Fried" Catfish

*Makes 4 servings * Per serving: 244 calories, 9 grams fat, 54 milligrams cholesterol, 86 milligrams sodium, 18 grams carbohydrate, 21 grams protein.*

Nonstick cooking spray

1/2 cup yellow cornmeal

2 tablespoons unbleached all-purpose flour

1 teaspoon chili powder

1/4 teaspoon paprika

1 teaspoon salt (optional)

1/4 teaspoon ground black pepper

1/4 cup evaporated skim milk

4 catfish fillets (about 1 pound)

Optional garnish: lemon wedges

Heat oven to 450°F. Spray broiler-pan rack with nonstick cooking spray. On sheet of waxed paper, mix cornmeal, flour, chili powder, paprika, salt and pepper until blended. Spread cornmeal mixture evenly on waxed paper or plate. Pour milk into shallow dish or pie plate. Dip a fillet in milk, covering completely. Dredge in cornmeal mixture until evenly coated. Place on broiler-pan rack. Coat remaining fillets; arrange on rack without them touching. Lightly spritz with cooking spray (to add to browning and crispiness). Bake, uncovered, until fish is cooked through and flakes easily when tested with fork, about 15 minutes. Garnish with lemon wedges.

Guide to Olive Oils (continued)

acidity. The olives are possibly of a lower quality. Use as an all-purpose oil that adds mild flavor to sautéing and stir-frying.

3. Pure Olive Oil (often simply labeled "olive oil") is extracted from the pulp left after making extra virgin oil. It's the least expensive yet quite suitable, especially for frying, as it has a high smoke-point.

4. Extra Light Olive Oil refers only to color and flavor, and not to the number of calories, which is the same as other olive oils (all have 120 calories per tablespoon). The mild flavor makes this filtered oil a good choice for baking.

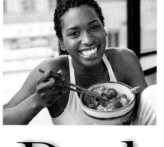

Nourish Your Body at Every Age

How old you are doesn't matter when it comes to loving life, but does when it comes to fueling your body. Use this guide to determine what you need most—and what foods to find it in—throughout your 20s, 30s, 40s, and 50s. »

Your 20s

No one is going to make you eat your veggies now, so you'll have to form your own good-nutrition habits. Put colorful foods on your plate and don't just buy whatever's cheap and easy.

Your special needs: Make sure you're getting at least 18 milligrams (mg) of iron a day. "Iron deficiency is the most common nutrient deficiency among women," says Jeannette Jordan, R.D., a Charleston, South Carolina–based registered dietitian. The signs: fatigue, lightheadedness, headaches, and cold hands and feet. Get your vitamin C (75 mg a day), which improves the absorption of iron. And don't skimp on two to three daily servings (1,000 mg) of calcium for strong bones and teeth. And all women of childbearing age must include 400 mg of folate daily for healthy development of babies in early pregnancy.

Your 30s

Managing a growing family? Grabbing a quick lunch between meetings? Eating healthfully when you're taking care of business is critical to keep your energy up.

Your special needs: Your metabolism may be changing, so watch calories more closely and beware of your risks for hypertension and diabetes. "Limit sodium, excess sugar and empty calories like soda," Lisa Young, Ph.D., R.D., adjunct professor of nutrition at New York University. Got babies on the brain? Be sure you're getting your 400 mg of folate daily (600 mg if you're pregnant) for healthy little ones. You'll also want to check your iron intake: If you're pregnant you need 27 mg a day, and if you're nursing, you need at least 9 mg a day. Getting enough vitamin C helps with iron absorption, and magnesium can ease PMS. »

Your 40s

You've got your weekly menus down to a science, but make sure to adjust for your changing metabolism, especially as you enter perimenopause.

Your special needs: In perimenopause, your risks rise for heart disease and diabetes. Get your calcium (1,000 mg a day) to counter bone loss. Be sure you're getting enough vitamin D and magnesium, which help your body absorb and use the calcium. You may need to adjust your fiber intake (at least 25 grams a day) to counter constipation and help reduce risk of heart disease, and potassium (4,700 mg a day) to help maintain a healthy blood pressure. Omega-3 fatty acid's inflammation-fighting properties can also reduce the risk of heart disease. Reduce your sodium to less than 2,300 mg daily to reduce your risk of hypertension.

Your 50s

You may look 40, but don't let the mirror fool you. Menopause brings radical changes your diet needs to respond to.

Your special needs: As estrogen declines, you're at greater risk for osteoporosis and heart disease. You need at least 1,200 mg of calcium a day to make up for bone loss if you're not on estrogen therapy. Vitamin D and magnesium help your body absorb and use the calcium, but you're at particular risk for vitamin D deficiency because older skin cannot process vitamin D as efficiently and darker skin is less able to produce vitamin D from sunlight. Experts are studying the role of magnesium, which helps regulate blood sugar levels and promotes normal blood pressure, in preventing disorders like hypertension, heart disease and diabetes. Get your B's: Macronutrients like vitamins B6 (1.5 mg/day) and B12 (2.4 mg/day) help fight hardening of the arteries.

Get Your Nutrients Here...

Calcium: Milk (use lactose-free or soy products if you need to), cheese, yogurt, broccoli, kale, corn tortillas, fortified products like orange juice. Ask your doc about calcium supplements that include vitamin D.

Fiber: Whole grains (oats, wheat, brown rice, rye, corn), black-eyed peas, black beans, lima beans, kidney beans, navy beans, chick peas, lentils, split peas. **Folate:** Fortified cereals, whole-grain breads, dark, leafy veg-etables, black-eyed peas. **Iron:** Red meats, fortified cere-als, egg yolks, beans, peas, green leafy vegetables. **Magnesium:** Fish like halibut, green veg-etables, beans, potatoes, nuts, seeds, whole, unrefined grains.

Omega-3s: Fish oils, some plant and nut oils. **Potassium:** Sweet potatoes, white potatoes, tomato paste, lima beans, car-rot juice, greens, prune juice. **Vitamin B6:** Bananas, pota-toes, pomegran-ates, fortified cereals.

Vitamin B12: Eggs, fish, chicken, meat, fortified cereals. **Vitamin C:** Citrus fruits, tomatoes, po-tatoes, brussel sprouts, straw-berries, cab-bage, spinach. **Vitamin D:** Fish liver oils, liver, fortified milk and cereals.

Menopause Symptoms: Plant-based supplements like black cohosh and dong quai are recommended by some ex-perts for hot flashes and other symp-toms. Consult with your doctor first.

Part 6:
Healthy Living Journal

Start Your Journey }

Ready to write down your goals and track your progress toward better health?

Use the first pages of this journal to create a picture of what the new you looks like, whether she's someone focused on working exercise into her schedule to slim down or eager to eat more healthfully to feel good. Then record your activity in the subsequent pages—or copy blank pages to write in—to help you stay the course and make your dream real! »

Personalized Food + Fitness Plan

Respond to the following questions to come up with a
plan of action for healthier living that works for *you*. »

MY MOTIVATION

1) How will I and my loved ones benefit from the changes I am making in my life? What is my greatest motivation?

_____

_____

_____

_____

MY FOOD PLAN

2) What negative thoughts have I had about food? What new ideas will I adopt to replace those negative thoughts?

_____

_____

_____

_____

3) What specific approach to healthier eating will work for me (for example, join a weight-loss program, leave high-calorie snacks on the supermarket shelf, use fitter recipes, bring a bag lunch to the office, keep a food diary, etc.)?

_____

_____

4) How many calories per day will I consume? _____

5) What are some good food choices for:

Breakfast: _____

Lunch: _____

Dinner: _____

Snacks: _____

6) What setbacks might I face? What strategies can I use to meet these situations?

_____

7) What nonfood rewards will I give myself to celebrate my small and large successes?

_____

MY EXERCISE PLAN

8) What kinds of exercise do I most enjoy? How can I work them into my plan?

Cardio: _____

Strength: _____

Flexibility: _____

9) When, where and for how long will I work out? How many times per week?

_____

_____

10) What is my exercise contingency plan in case the weather is bad/ my workload gets insane/ I am traveling?

_____

_____

11) How will I keep things interesting and fun?

_____

_____

12) What is my greatest challenge, and how will I address it?

_____

_____

13) Where else can I incorporate activity into my life? (For example, get a pedometer and count 12,000 to 15,000 steps each day, walk to the store instead of driving, take up gardening, use the stairs, etc.)

_____

_____

MY SUPPORT SYSTEM

14) Whom will I enlist to join my cheering squad (for example, a nutritionist, trainer, therapist, weekly support group, friends, family members, coworkers, etc.)?

_____

_____

15) What is the best way for a friend or family member to support me?

_____

_____

16) If I lose motivation or focus, what three positive thoughts and actions will I embrace to get back on track?

_____

_____

DATE:

_____

HOURS
OF SLEEP:

_____

HOW
STRESSED
ARE YOU
TODAY? (1-10)

_____

WHAT YOU DID
TO UNWIND:

_____

_____

_____

WHAT'S YOUR
HEALTH GOAL
FOR THE DAY?:

_____

WEIGHT:

_____

BMI:

_____

BEDTIME:

_____

Food Log:

Breakfast: _____
_____
_____
Lunch: _____
_____
_____
Dinner: _____
_____
_____
Beverages: _____
_____
Snacks: _____

Notes:

_____
_____
_____
_____
_____
_____
_____
_____
_____
_____
_____

Exercise Log:

Cardio: _____ Time: _____
Distance: _____ Level: _____

Flexibility: _____
Stretches: _____
Classes: _____

Strength: _____ Weight: _____
Repetitions: _____ Sets: _____

Notes: _____
_____
_____

DATE:

_____

**HOURS
OF SLEEP:**

_____

**HOW
STRESSED
ARE YOU
TODAY? (1-10)**

_____

**WHAT YOU DID
TO UNWIND:**

_____

_____

**WHAT'S YOUR
HEALTH GOAL
FOR THE DAY?**

_____

WEIGHT:

_____

BMI:

_____

BEDTIME:

_____

Food Log:

Breakfast: _____
_____
_____

Lunch: _____
_____
_____

Dinner: _____
_____
_____

Beverages: _____
_____

Snacks: _____

Notes:

_____
_____
_____
_____
_____
_____
_____
_____
_____
_____

Exercise Log:

Cardio: _____   Time: _____
Distance: _____   Level: _____

Flexibility: _____
Stretches: _____
Classes: _____

Strength: _____   Weight: _____
Repetitions: _____   Sets: _____

✱Feel Stronger Now! Want to pick up your child with ease, cart the groceries without feeling it the next day, and do yard work in one wave? Work push-ups into your exercise routine. Here's what you should aim for:

If you're in your 20s: **12–22 push-ups**	If you're in your 30s: **10–21 push-ups**
If you're in your 40s: **8–17 push-ups**	If you're in your 50s: **7–14 push-ups**

DATE:
_____

HOURS
OF SLEEP:
_____

HOW
STRESSED
ARE YOU
TODAY? (1-10)
_____

WHAT YOU DID
TO UNWIND:
_____
_____
_____

WHAT'S YOUR
HEALTH GOAL
FOR THE DAY?:
_____

WEIGHT:
_____

BMI:
_____

BEDTIME:
_____

Food Log:

Breakfast: _____
_____
_____

Lunch: _____
_____
_____

Dinner: _____
_____
_____

Beverages: _____
_____

Snacks: _____

Notes:
_____
_____
_____
_____
_____
_____
_____
_____
_____
_____

Exercise Log:

Cardio: _____   Time: _____
Distance: _____   Level: _____

Flexibility: _____
Stretches: _____
Classes: _____

Strength: _____   Weight: _____
Repetitions: _____ Sets: _____

Notes: _____
_____
_____

DATE:

_____

**HOURS
OF SLEEP:**

_____

**HOW
STRESSED
ARE YOU
TODAY? (1-10)**

_____

**WHAT YOU DID
TO UNWIND:**

_____

_____

**WHAT'S YOUR
HEALTH GOAL
FOR THE DAY?**

_____

WEIGHT:

_____

BMI:

_____

BEDTIME:

_____

Food Log:

Breakfast: _____

_____

_____

Lunch: _____

_____

_____

Dinner: _____

_____

_____

Beverages: _____

Snacks: _____

Notes:

_____

_____

_____

_____

_____

_____

_____

_____

_____

Exercise Log:

Cardio: _____   Time: _____

Distance: _____   Level: _____

Flexibility: _____

Stretches: _____

Classes: _____

Strength: _____   Weight: _____

Repetitions: _____   Sets: _____

✷**Shrink Your Order.** "Instead of the three-piece meal, get the two-piece," says Nelson L. Adams, president of the National Medical Association and chair of the obstetrics and gynecology department at Jackson North Medical Center in Miami, Florida. If you normally order a regular cheeseburger, get the junior size.

DATE:

_____

HOURS
OF SLEEP:

_____

HOW
STRESSED
ARE YOU
TODAY? (1-10)

_____

WHAT YOU DID
TO UNWIND:

_____

_____

_____

WHAT'S YOUR
HEALTH GOAL
FOR THE DAY?:

_____

WEIGHT:

_____

BMI:

_____

BEDTIME:

_____

Food Log:

Breakfast: _____
_____
_____
Lunch: _____
_____
_____
Dinner: _____
_____
_____
Beverages: _____
_____
Snacks: _____

Notes:

_____
_____
_____
_____
_____
_____
_____
_____
_____
_____
_____

Exercise Log:

Cardio: _____ Time: _____
Distance: _____ Level: _____

Flexibility: _____
Stretches: _____
Classes: _____

Strength: _____ Weight: _____
Repetitions: _____ Sets: _____

Notes: _____
_____
_____

DATE:

_____

**HOURS
OF SLEEP:**

_____

**HOW
STRESSED
ARE YOU
TODAY? (1-10)**

_____

**WHAT YOU DID
TO UNWIND:**

_____

_____

_____

**WHAT'S YOUR
HEALTH GOAL
FOR THE DAY?**

_____

_____

WEIGHT:

_____

BMI:

_____

BEDTIME:

_____

Food Log:

Breakfast: _____
_____
_____

Lunch: _____
_____
_____

Dinner: _____
_____
_____

Beverages: _____
_____

Snacks: _____

Notes:

_____
_____
_____
_____
_____
_____
_____
_____
_____
_____
_____

Exercise Log:

Cardio: _____   Time: _____
Distance: _____   Level: _____

Flexibility: _____
Stretches: _____
Classes: _____

Strength: _____   Weight: _____
Repetitions: _____   Sets: _____

✱Quit Hitting Snooze. Those 5-minute catnaps you create by tapping your alarm clock don't allow you to go far enough into deep sleep. "What you're really doing is stealing sleep, which can cause you to become chronically sleep deprived," says Timothy Collins, M.D., a pulmonologist with the Kaiser Permanente Colorado.

DATE:
_____

HOURS
OF SLEEP:
_____

HOW
STRESSED
ARE YOU
TODAY? (1-10)
_____

WHAT YOU DID
TO UNWIND:
_____
_____
_____

WHAT'S YOUR
HEALTH GOAL
FOR THE DAY?:
_____

WEIGHT:
_____

BMI:
_____

BEDTIME:
_____

Food Log:

Breakfast: _____
_____
_____

Lunch: _____
_____
_____

Dinner: _____
_____
_____

Beverages: _____
_____

Snacks: _____

Notes:
_____
_____
_____
_____
_____
_____
_____
_____
_____
_____

Exercise Log:

Cardio: _____   Time: _____

Distance: _____   Level: _____

Flexibility: _____

Stretches: _____

Classes: _____

Strength: _____   Weight: _____

Repetitions: _____   Sets: _____

Notes: _____
_____
_____

DATE:

_____

**HOURS
OF SLEEP:**

_____

**HOW
STRESSED
ARE YOU
TODAY? (1-10)**

_____

**WHAT YOU DID
TO UNWIND:**

_____

_____

_____

**WHAT'S YOUR
HEALTH GOAL
FOR THE DAY?**

_____

WEIGHT:

_____

BMI:

_____

BEDTIME:

_____

Food Log:

Breakfast: _____

_____

_____

Lunch: _____

_____

_____

Dinner: _____

_____

_____

Beverages: _____

_____

Snacks: _____

Notes:

_____

_____

_____

_____

_____

_____

_____

_____

_____

_____

_____

_____

Exercise Log:

Cardio: _____   Time: _____

Distance: _____   Level: _____

Flexibility: _____

Stretches: _____

Classes: _____

Strength: _____   Weight: _____

Repetitions: _____   Sets: _____

✳ What to Eat Today? Consult the USDA's customizable Food Pyramid at mypyramid.gov. It says, for example, a 38-year-old woman who's 5'5", 145 pounds and works out less than 30 minutes a day needs 2.5 cups of vegetables, 2 cups of fruits, 3 cups of milk and 5.5 ounces of meat.

DATE:

_____

HOURS
OF SLEEP:

_____

HOW
STRESSED
ARE YOU
TODAY? (1-10)

_____

WHAT YOU DID
TO UNWIND:

_____

_____

_____

WHAT'S YOUR
HEALTH GOAL
FOR THE DAY?:

_____

WEIGHT:

_____

BMI:

_____

BEDTIME:

_____

Food Log:

Breakfast: _____
_____
_____

Lunch: _____
_____
_____

Dinner: _____
_____
_____

Beverages: _____
_____

Snacks: _____

Notes:

_____
_____
_____
_____
_____
_____
_____
_____
_____
_____

Exercise Log:

Cardio: _____   Time: _____
Distance: _____   Level: _____

Flexibility: _____
Stretches: _____
Classes: _____

Strength: _____   Weight: _____
Repetitions: _____   Sets: _____

Notes: _____
_____
_____

DATE:

_____

HOURS OF SLEEP:

_____

HOW STRESSED ARE YOU TODAY? (1-10)

_____

WHAT YOU DID TO UNWIND:

_____

_____

_____

WHAT'S YOUR HEALTH GOAL FOR THE DAY?

_____

WEIGHT:

_____

BMI:

_____

BEDTIME:

_____

Food Log:

Breakfast: _____

_____

_____

Lunch: _____

_____

_____

Dinner: _____

_____

_____

Beverages: _____

_____

Snacks: _____

Notes:

_____

_____

_____

_____

_____

_____

_____

_____

_____

_____

_____

Exercise Log:

Cardio: _____   Time: _____

Distance: _____   Level: _____

Flexibility: _____

Stretches: _____

Classes: _____

Strength: _____   Weight: _____

Repetitions: _____   Sets: _____

✳ Get Your Heart Racing. While any level of exercise can help lower stress, research has shown that high-intensity activities may do so better. Going for a run? Consider doing sprint intervals or a hilly course. About to hit a step aerobics class? Try doubling up on your risers.

DATE:

_____

HOURS
OF SLEEP:

_____

HOW
STRESSED
ARE YOU
TODAY? (1-10)

_____

WHAT YOU DID
TO UNWIND:

_____

_____

_____

WHAT'S YOUR
HEALTH GOAL
FOR THE DAY?:

_____

WEIGHT:

_____

BMI:

_____

BEDTIME:

_____

Food Log:

Breakfast: _____

_____

_____

Lunch: _____

_____

_____

Dinner: _____

_____

_____

Beverages: _____

_____

Snacks: _____

Notes:

_____

_____

_____

_____

_____

_____

_____

_____

_____

_____

_____

Exercise Log:

Cardio: _____   Time: _____

Distance: _____   Level: _____

Flexibility: _____

Stretches: _____

Classes: _____

Strength: _____   Weight: _____

Repetitions: _____   Sets: _____

Notes: _____

_____

_____

DATE:

_____

**HOURS
OF SLEEP:**

_____

**HOW
STRESSED
ARE YOU
TODAY? (1-10)**

_____

**WHAT YOU DID
TO UNWIND:**

_____

_____

_____

**WHAT'S YOUR
HEALTH GOAL
FOR THE DAY?**

_____

WEIGHT:

_____

BMI:

_____

BEDTIME:

_____

Food Log:

Breakfast: _____

_____

_____

Lunch: _____

_____

_____

Dinner: _____

_____

_____

Beverages: _____

_____

Snacks: _____

Notes:

_____

_____

_____

_____

_____

_____

_____

_____

_____

Exercise Log:

Cardio: _____   Time: _____

Distance: _____   Level: _____

Flexibility: _____

Stretches: _____

Classes: _____

Strength: _____   Weight: _____

Repetitions: _____   Sets: _____

✳**Make Yourself a Priority.** "I've found that if I make time for what I enjoy the most, like time with my family or exercise, I'm more efficient at work," says Andrea Pennington, M.D., coauthor of _The Pennington Plan: 5 Simple Steps for Achieving Vibrant Health, Emotional Well-Being and Spiritual Growth_ (Avery).

DATE:

_____

HOURS
OF SLEEP:

_____

HOW
STRESSED
ARE YOU
TODAY? (1-10)

_____

WHAT YOU DID
TO UNWIND:

_____

_____

_____

WHAT'S YOUR
HEALTH GOAL
FOR THE DAY?:

_____

WEIGHT:

_____

BMI:

_____

BEDTIME:

_____

Food Log:

Breakfast: _____

_____

_____

Lunch: _____

_____

_____

Dinner: _____

_____

_____

Beverages: _____

_____

Snacks: _____

Notes:

_____

_____

_____

_____

_____

_____

_____

_____

_____

_____

Exercise Log:

Cardio: _____ Time: _____
Distance: _____ Level: _____

Flexibility: _____
Stretches: _____
Classes: _____

Strength: _____ Weight: _____
Repetitions: _____ Sets: _____

Notes: _____

_____

_____

DATE:

_____

**HOURS
OF SLEEP:**

_____

**HOW
STRESSED
ARE YOU
TODAY? (1-10)**

_____

**WHAT YOU DID
TO UNWIND:**

_____

_____

_____

**WHAT'S YOUR
HEALTH GOAL
FOR THE DAY?:**

_____

WEIGHT:

_____

BMI:

_____

BEDTIME:

_____

Food Log:

Breakfast: _____
_____
_____

Lunch: _____
_____
_____

Dinner: _____
_____
_____

Beverages: _____
_____

Snacks: _____

Notes:

_____
_____
_____
_____
_____
_____
_____
_____
_____

Exercise Log:

Cardio: _____   Time: _____
Distance: _____   Level: _____

Flexibility: _____
Stretches: _____
Classes: _____

Strength: _____   Weight: _____
Repetitions: _____ Sets: _____

✳ Schedule Free Time. It's important to have goals, but one of them should be to master the art of unwinding. "Do nothing for at least a few minutes a day," says Valorie Burton, author of _What's Really Holding You Back?_ (WaterBrook). "It's one of the best ways to decrease your stress level."

DATE:

_____

**HOURS
OF SLEEP:**

_____

**HOW
STRESSED
ARE YOU
TODAY? (1-10)**

_____

**WHAT YOU DID
TO UNWIND:**

_____

_____

_____

**WHAT'S YOUR
HEALTH GOAL
FOR THE DAY?:**

_____

WEIGHT:

_____

BMI:

_____

BEDTIME:

_____

Food Log:

Breakfast: _____
_____
_____

Lunch: _____
_____
_____

Dinner: _____
_____
_____

Beverages: _____
_____

Snacks: _____

Notes:

_____
_____
_____
_____
_____
_____
_____
_____
_____
_____

Exercise Log:

Cardio: _____   Time: _____
Distance: _____   Level: _____

Flexibility: _____
Stretches: _____
Classes: _____

Strength: _____   Weight: _____
Repetitions: _____   Sets: _____

Notes: _____
_____

DATE:

_____

**HOURS
OF SLEEP:**

_____

**HOW
STRESSED
ARE YOU
TODAY? (1-10)**

_____

**WHAT YOU DID
TO UNWIND:**

_____

_____

_____

**WHAT'S YOUR
HEALTH GOAL
FOR THE DAY?:**

_____

WEIGHT:

_____

BMI:

_____

BEDTIME:

_____

Food Log:

Breakfast: _____

_____

_____

Lunch: _____

_____

_____

Dinner: _____

_____

_____

Beverages: _____

Snacks: _____

Notes:

_____

_____

_____

_____

_____

_____

_____

_____

_____

Exercise Log:

Cardio: _____   Time: _____

Distance: _____   Level: _____

Flexibility: _____

Stretches: _____

Classes: _____

Strength: _____   Weight: _____

Repetitions: _____   Sets: _____

＊Love Your Legs. Try this squat extension from Rossalyn Quaye Fischer, membership adviser at Equinox
Fitness Club and former trainer: Begin in squat position with arms straight in front of you. As you stand, shift weight
onto left leg, extend right leg behind you, and flex right foot. At the same time, turn palms upward, clench fists,
and pull hands to sides of waist. Return to starting position. Repeat exercise on opposite side. Do ten to 15 reps.

DATE:

_____

HOURS
OF SLEEP:

_____

HOW
STRESSED
ARE YOU
TODAY? (1-10)

_____

WHAT YOU DID
TO UNWIND:

_____

_____

_____

WHAT'S YOUR
HEALTH GOAL
FOR THE DAY?:

_____

WEIGHT:

_____

BMI:

_____

BEDTIME:

_____

Food Log:

Breakfast: _____
_____
_____

Lunch: _____
_____

Dinner: _____
_____

Beverages: _____
_____

Snacks: _____

Notes:

_____
_____
_____
_____
_____
_____
_____
_____
_____
_____
_____
_____

Exercise Log:

Cardio: _____   Time: _____
Distance: _____   Level: _____

Flexibility: _____
Stretches: _____
Classes: _____

Strength: _____   Weight: _____
Repetitions: _____   Sets: _____

Notes: _____
_____
_____

DATE:
_____

HOURS OF SLEEP:
_____

HOW STRESSED ARE YOU TODAY? (1-10)
_____

WHAT YOU DID TO UNWIND:
_____
_____
_____

WHAT'S YOUR HEALTH GOAL FOR THE DAY?:
_____

WEIGHT:
_____

BMI:
_____

BEDTIME:
_____

Food Log:

Breakfast: _____
_____
_____

Lunch: _____
_____
_____

Dinner: _____
_____
_____

Beverages: _____
_____

Snacks: _____

Notes:
_____
_____
_____
_____
_____
_____
_____
_____

Exercise Log:

Cardio: _____ Time: _____
Distance: _____ Level: _____

Flexibility: _____
Stretches: _____
Classes: _____

Strength: _____ Weight: _____
Repetitions: _____ Sets: _____

✱ Trick Your Eyes. "Studies show that if you have smaller plate, you eat smaller portions," say Jonny Bowden, Ph.D., C.N.S., a board-certified nutrition specialist and author of *The Most Effective Natural Cures on Earth* (Fair Winds Press). "Appreciation and satisfaction are deeply rooted in the visual and subconscious."

DATE:

_____

**HOURS
OF SLEEP:**

_____

**HOW
STRESSED
ARE YOU
TODAY? (1-10)**

_____

**WHAT YOU DID
TO UNWIND:**

_____

_____

_____

**WHAT'S YOUR
HEALTH GOAL
FOR THE DAY?:**

_____

WEIGHT:

_____

BMI:

_____

BEDTIME:

_____

Food Log:

Breakfast: _____

_____

_____

Lunch: _____

_____

_____

Dinner: _____

_____

_____

Beverages: _____

_____

Snacks: _____

Notes:

_____

_____

_____

_____

_____

_____

_____

_____

_____

_____

_____

Exercise Log:

Cardio: _____ Time: _____
Distance: _____ Level: _____

Flexibility: _____
Stretches: _____
Classes: _____

Strength: _____ Weight: _____
Repetitions: _____ Sets: _____

Notes: _____

_____

_____

DATE:

_____

HOURS OF SLEEP:

_____

HOW STRESSED ARE YOU TODAY? (1-10)

_____

WHAT YOU DID TO UNWIND:

_____

_____

_____

WHAT'S YOUR HEALTH GOAL FOR THE DAY?:

_____

WEIGHT:

_____

BMI:

_____

BEDTIME:

_____

Food Log:

Breakfast: _____

_____

_____

Lunch: _____

_____

_____

Dinner: _____

_____

_____

Beverages: _____

_____

Snacks: _____

Notes:

_____

_____

_____

_____

_____

_____

_____

_____

_____

_____

_____

Exercise Log:

Cardio: _____ Time: _____

Distance: _____ Level: _____

Flexibility: _____

Stretches: _____

Classes: _____

Strength: _____ Weight: _____

Repetitions: _____ Sets: _____

* **Think "Activity" Rather Than "Workout."** Focus on playing tag with your kids, vacuuming, hitting a tennis ball back and forth, dancing, and walking around a track or park with friends. All those activities count as exercise. Even ten-minute increments can strengthen your heart and boost your emotions.

DATE:

_____

HOURS
OF SLEEP:

_____

HOW
STRESSED
ARE YOU
TODAY? (1-10)

_____

WHAT YOU DID
TO UNWIND:

_____

_____

_____

WHAT'S YOUR
HEALTH GOAL
FOR THE DAY?:

_____

WEIGHT:

_____

BMI:

_____

BEDTIME:

_____

Food Log:

Breakfast: _____

_____

_____

Lunch: _____

_____

_____

Dinner: _____

_____

_____

Beverages: _____

_____

Snacks: _____

Notes:

_____

_____

_____

_____

_____

_____

_____

_____

_____

_____

_____

Exercise Log:

Cardio: _____   Time: _____
Distance: _____   Level: _____

Flexibility: _____
Stretches: _____
Classes: _____

Strength: _____   Weight: _____
Repetitions: _____   Sets: _____

Notes: _____

_____

_____

DATE:

_____

**HOURS
OF SLEEP:**

_____

**HOW
STRESSED
ARE YOU
TODAY? (1-10)**

_____

**WHAT YOU DID
TO UNWIND:**

_____

_____

_____

**WHAT'S YOUR
HEALTH GOAL
FOR THE DAY?:**

_____

WEIGHT:

_____

BMI:

_____

BEDTIME:

_____

Food Log:

Breakfast: _____

_____

_____

Lunch: _____

_____

_____

Dinner: _____

_____

_____

Beverages: _____

Snacks: _____

Notes:

_____

_____

_____

_____

_____

_____

_____

_____

_____

_____

_____

Exercise Log:

Cardio: _____   Time: _____
Distance: _____   Level: _____

Flexibility: _____
Stretches: _____
Classes: _____

Strength: _____   Weight: _____
Repetitions: _____   Sets: _____

✱Be Willing to Start Over. If you skip the gym one day or supersize lunch one afternoon, don't give up! The temptation may be to throw in the towel and indulge yourself all day (or week) long. But the smarter solution? Say 'I screwed up,' then get back on track for your next meal or workout.

DATE:

_____

HOURS OF SLEEP:

_____

HOW STRESSED ARE YOU TODAY? (1-10)

_____

WHAT YOU DID TO UNWIND:

_____

_____

_____

WHAT'S YOUR HEALTH GOAL FOR THE DAY?:

_____

WEIGHT:

_____

BMI:

_____

BEDTIME:

_____

Food Log:

Breakfast: _____

_____

_____

Lunch: _____

_____

_____

Dinner: _____

_____

_____

Beverages: _____

_____

Snacks: _____

Notes:

_____

_____

_____

_____

_____

_____

_____

_____

_____

_____

Exercise Log:

Cardio: _____ Time: _____
Distance: _____ Level: _____

Flexibility: _____
Stretches: _____
Classes: _____

Strength: _____ Weight: _____
Repetitions: _____ Sets: _____

Notes: _____

_____

_____

DATE:

_____

**HOURS
OF SLEEP:**

_____

**HOW
STRESSED
ARE YOU
TODAY? (1-10)**

_____

**WHAT YOU DID
TO UNWIND:**

_____

_____

_____

**WHAT'S YOUR
HEALTH GOAL
FOR THE DAY?:**

_____

WEIGHT:

_____

BMI:

_____

BEDTIME:

_____

Food Log:

Breakfast: _____

_____

_____

Lunch: _____

_____

_____

Dinner: _____

_____

_____

Beverages: _____

_____

Snacks: _____

Notes:

_____

_____

_____

_____

_____

_____

_____

_____

_____

_____

Exercise Log:

Cardio: _____   Time: _____
Distance: _____   Level: _____

Flexibility: _____
Stretches: _____
Classes: _____

Strength: _____   Weight: _____
Repetitions: _____   Sets: _____

✳ **Divide to Conquer.** Split desserts with friends, get half your meal to go, and separate sauces. "If you don't ask for your dressing on the side, you won't be able to monitor how much you're eating," says Lisa R. Young, Ph.D., R.D., adjunct professor of nutrition at New York University and author of _The Portion Teller Plan_ (Broadway).

DATE:

_____

HOURS
OF SLEEP:

_____

HOW
STRESSED
ARE YOU
TODAY? (1-10)

_____

WHAT YOU DID
TO UNWIND:

_____

_____

_____

WHAT'S YOUR
HEALTH GOAL
FOR THE DAY?:

_____

WEIGHT:

_____

BMI:

_____

BEDTIME:

_____

Food Log:

Breakfast: _____

_____

_____

Lunch: _____

_____

_____

Dinner: _____

_____

_____

Beverages: _____

_____

Snacks: _____

Notes:

_____

_____

_____

_____

_____

_____

_____

_____

_____

_____

_____

Exercise Log:

Cardio: _____   Time: _____
Distance: _____   Level: _____

Flexibility: _____
Stretches: _____
Classes: _____

Strength: _____   Weight: _____
Repetitions: _____   Sets: _____

Notes: _____

_____

_____

DATE:

_____

**HOURS
OF SLEEP:**

_____

**HOW
STRESSED
ARE YOU
TODAY? (1-10)**

_____

**WHAT YOU DID
TO UNWIND:**

_____

_____

_____

**WHAT'S YOUR
HEALTH GOAL
FOR THE DAY?:**

_____

WEIGHT:

_____

BMI:

_____

BEDTIME:

_____

Food Log:

Breakfast: _____

_____

_____

Lunch: _____

_____

_____

Dinner: _____

_____

_____

Beverages: _____

_____

Snacks: _____

Notes:

_____
_____
_____
_____
_____
_____
_____
_____
_____
_____
_____
_____

Exercise Log:

Cardio: _____ Time: _____
Distance: _____ Level: _____

Flexibility: _____
Stretches: _____
Classes: _____

Strength: _____ Weight: _____
Repetitions: _____ Sets: _____

✳ Breathe in Relaxation. Studies show a connection between the nose and memory, which means you can train your brain to think of sleep with the whiff of a relaxing bedtime scent of your choice. For all-night aromatherapy, use a linen spray or your favorite body lotion in calming scents like lavender and chamomile.

DATE:

_____

HOURS
OF SLEEP:

_____

HOW
STRESSED
ARE YOU
TODAY? (1-10)

_____

WHAT YOU DID
TO UNWIND:

_____

_____

_____

WHAT'S YOUR
HEALTH GOAL
FOR THE DAY?:

_____

WEIGHT:

_____

BMI:

_____

BEDTIME:

_____

Food Log:

Breakfast: _____
_____
_____

Lunch: _____
_____
_____

Dinner: _____
_____
_____

Beverages: _____
_____

Snacks: _____

Notes:

_____
_____
_____
_____
_____
_____
_____
_____
_____
_____

Exercise Log:

Cardio: _____   Time: _____
Distance: _____   Level: _____

Flexibility: _____
Stretches: _____
Classes: _____

Strength: _____   Weight: _____
Repetitions: _____   Sets: _____

Notes: _____
_____
_____

DATE:

_____

**HOURS
OF SLEEP:**

_____

**HOW
STRESSED
ARE YOU
TODAY? (1-10)**

_____

**WHAT YOU DID
TO UNWIND:**

_____

_____

_____

**WHAT'S YOUR
HEALTH GOAL
FOR THE DAY?:**

_____

WEIGHT:

_____

BMI:

_____

BEDTIME:

_____

Food Log:

Breakfast: _____

_____

_____

Lunch: _____

_____

_____

Dinner: _____

_____

_____

Beverages: _____

_____

Snacks: _____

Notes:

_____

_____

_____

_____

_____

_____

_____

_____

_____

_____

Exercise Log:

Cardio: _____ Time: _____

Distance: _____ Level: _____

Flexibility: _____

Stretches: _____

Classes: _____

Strength: _____ Weight: _____

Repetitions: _____ Sets: _____

✳Keep a Bliss List. For one week, rate every activity you engage in by how much pleasure it gives you, and figure out how to work more of the high rankers into your day. You may find a ten-minute quickie with your man helps you de-stress better than an hour zoned out in front of the TV.

DATE:

_____

**HOURS
OF SLEEP:**

_____

**HOW
STRESSED
ARE YOU
TODAY? (1-10)**

_____

**WHAT YOU DID
TO UNWIND:**

_____

_____

_____

**WHAT'S YOUR
HEALTH GOAL
FOR THE DAY?:**

_____

WEIGHT:

_____

BMI:

_____

BEDTIME:

_____

Food Log:

Breakfast: _____

_____

Lunch: _____

_____

_____

Dinner: _____

_____

_____

Beverages: _____

_____

Snacks: _____

Notes:

_____

_____

_____

_____

_____

_____

_____

_____

_____

_____

Exercise Log:

Cardio: _____   Time: _____
Distance: _____   Level: _____

Flexibility: _____
Stretches: _____
Classes: _____

Strength: _____   Weight: _____
Repetitions: _____   Sets: _____

Notes: _____

_____

_____

DATE:

_____

**HOURS
OF SLEEP:**

_____

**HOW
STRESSED
ARE YOU
TODAY? (1-10)**

_____

**WHAT YOU DID
TO UNWIND:**

_____

_____

_____

**WHAT'S YOUR
HEALTH GOAL
FOR THE DAY?:**

_____

WEIGHT:

_____

BMI:

_____

BEDTIME:

_____

Food Log:

Breakfast: _____

_____

_____

Lunch: _____

_____

_____

Dinner: _____

_____

_____

Beverages: _____

_____

Snacks: _____

Notes:

_____

_____

_____

_____

_____

_____

_____

_____

_____

_____

_____

Exercise Log:

Cardio: _____ Time: _____
Distance: _____ Level: _____

Flexibility: _____
Stretches: _____
Classes: _____

Strength: _____ Weight: _____
Repetitions: _____ Sets: _____

✳ Lose Love Handles. Try this move from Rossalyn Quaye Fischer, membership adviser at Equinox Fitness Club and former trainer: Lie on your back, point arms in front of you, lift knees to a 90-degree angle and torso to 45 degrees. With palms facing downward, bring hands to chest so fingertips touch and elbows point out. Turn torso left and tap the floor with left hand. Return to center. Repeat on right with right arm. Do ten reps.

DATE:

_____

HOURS
OF SLEEP:

_____

HOW
STRESSED
ARE YOU
TODAY? (1-10)

_____

WHAT YOU DID
TO UNWIND:

_____

_____

_____

WHAT'S YOUR
HEALTH GOAL
FOR THE DAY?:

_____

WEIGHT:

_____

BMI:

_____

BEDTIME:

_____

Food Log:

Breakfast: _____
_____
_____

Lunch: _____
_____
_____

Dinner: _____
_____
_____

Beverages: _____
_____

Snacks: _____

Notes:

_____
_____
_____
_____
_____
_____
_____
_____
_____

Exercise Log:

Cardio: _____   Time: _____
Distance: _____   Level: _____

Flexibility: _____
Stretches: _____
Classes: _____

Strength: _____   Weight: _____
Repetitions: _____   Sets: _____

Notes: _____
_____
_____

DATE:

_____

**HOURS
OF SLEEP:**

_____

**HOW
STRESSED
ARE YOU
TODAY? (1-10)**

_____

**WHAT YOU DID
TO UNWIND:**

_____

_____

_____

**WHAT'S YOUR
HEALTH GOAL
FOR THE DAY?:**

_____

WEIGHT:

_____

BMI:

_____

BEDTIME:

_____

Food Log:

Breakfast: _____
_____
_____

Lunch: _____
_____
_____

Dinner: _____
_____
_____

Beverages: _____
_____

Snacks: _____

Notes:

_____
_____
_____
_____
_____
_____
_____
_____
_____
_____
_____

Exercise Log:

Cardio: _____   Time: _____
Distance: _____   Level: _____

Flexibility: _____
Stretches: _____
Classes: _____

Strength: _____   Weight: _____
Repetitions: _____   Sets: _____

❊ Prepare Your Own Food. "Most of the salt in a diet doesn't come from the salt shaker on your table, but from processed foods like canned soup," says Jonny Bowden, Ph.D., C.N.S., a board-certified nutrition specialist and author of _The Most Effective Natural Cures on Earth_ (Fair Winds Press).

DATE:

_____

HOURS
OF SLEEP:

_____

HOW
STRESSED
ARE YOU
TODAY? (1-10)

_____

WHAT YOU DID
TO UNWIND:

_____

_____

_____

WHAT'S YOUR
HEALTH GOAL
FOR THE DAY?:

_____

WEIGHT:

_____

BMI:

_____

BEDTIME:

_____

Food Log:

Breakfast: _____

_____

Lunch: _____

_____

Dinner: _____

_____

Beverages: _____

Snacks: _____

Notes:

_____

_____

_____

_____

_____

_____

_____

_____

_____

Exercise Log:

Cardio: _____   Time: _____
Distance: _____   Level: _____

Flexibility: _____
Stretches: _____
Classes: _____

Strength: _____   Weight: _____
Repetitions: _____   Sets: _____

Notes: _____

_____

_____

DATE:

_____

**HOURS
OF SLEEP:**

_____

**HOW
STRESSED
ARE YOU
TODAY? (1-10)**

_____

**WHAT YOU DID
TO UNWIND:**

_____

_____

**WHAT'S YOUR
HEALTH GOAL
FOR THE DAY?:**

_____

WEIGHT:

_____

BMI:

_____

BEDTIME:

_____

Food Log:

Breakfast: _____
_____
_____

Lunch: _____
_____
_____

Dinner: _____
_____
_____

Beverages: _____
_____

Snacks: _____

Notes:

_____
_____
_____
_____
_____
_____
_____
_____

Exercise Log:

Cardio: _____   Time: _____
Distance: _____   Level: _____

Flexibility: _____
Stretches: _____
Classes: _____

Strength: _____   Weight: _____
Repetitions: _____   Sets: _____

✱ Eat Consciously. "Ask yourself, _Am I eating this because I'm hungry or because it's here?_" says Lisa R. Young, Ph.D., R.D., adjunct professor of nutrition at New York University and author of _The Portion Teller Plan_ (Broadway). Turning in your membership card to the Clean Plate Club can free you of some excess calories.

DATE:

_____

HOURS
OF SLEEP:

_____

HOW
STRESSED
ARE YOU
TODAY? (1-10)

_____

WHAT YOU DID
TO UNWIND:

_____

_____

_____

WHAT'S YOUR
HEALTH GOAL
FOR THE DAY?:

_____

WEIGHT:

_____

BMI:

_____

BEDTIME:

_____

Food Log:

Breakfast: _____
_____
_____

Lunch: _____
_____
_____

Dinner: _____
_____
_____

Beverages: _____

Snacks: _____

Notes:

_____
_____
_____
_____
_____
_____
_____
_____
_____
_____

Exercise Log:

Cardio: _____   Time: _____
Distance: _____   Level: _____

Flexibility: _____
Stretches: _____
Classes: _____

Strength: _____   Weight: _____
Repetitions: _____   Sets: _____

Notes: _____
_____
_____

DATE:

_____

**HOURS
OF SLEEP:**

_____

**HOW
STRESSED
ARE YOU
TODAY? (1-10)**

_____

**WHAT YOU DID
TO UNWIND:**

_____

_____

**WHAT'S YOUR
HEALTH GOAL
FOR THE DAY?:**

_____

WEIGHT:

_____

BMI:

_____

BEDTIME:

_____

Food Log:

Breakfast: _____
_____
_____

Lunch: _____
_____
_____

Dinner: _____
_____
_____

Beverages: _____
_____

Snacks: _____

Notes:

_____
_____
_____
_____
_____
_____
_____
_____
_____
_____

Exercise Log:

Cardio: _____   Time: _____
Distance: _____   Level: _____

Flexibility: _____
Stretches: _____
Classes: _____

Strength: _____   Weight: _____
Repetitions: _____   Sets: _____

✳ **Reach for Sleep.** Can't drift off? Try this calming yoga move called child's pose: Kneel on your bed, sit back on your heels, and place a pillow or two between thighs. Stretch torso over pillows, letting your head rest on them and lengthening arms out in front of you. Relax and focus on breathing for 30 seconds to three minutes.

DATE:

_____

HOURS
OF SLEEP:

_____

HOW
STRESSED
ARE YOU
TODAY? (1-10)

_____

WHAT YOU DID
TO UNWIND:

_____

_____

_____

WHAT'S YOUR
HEALTH GOAL
FOR THE DAY?:

_____

WEIGHT:

_____

BMI:

_____

BEDTIME:

_____

Food Log:

Breakfast: _____

_____

_____

Lunch: _____

_____

_____

Dinner: _____

_____

_____

Beverages: _____

_____

Snacks: _____

Notes:

_____
_____
_____
_____
_____
_____
_____
_____
_____
_____
_____

Exercise Log:

Cardio: _____   Time: _____
Distance: _____   Level: _____

Flexibility: _____
Stretches: _____
Classes: _____

Strength: _____   Weight: _____
Repetitions: _____   Sets: _____

Notes: _____
_____
_____

DATE:

_____

**HOURS
OF SLEEP:**

_____

**HOW
STRESSED
ARE YOU
TODAY? (1-10)**

_____

**WHAT YOU DID
TO UNWIND:**

_____

_____

_____

**WHAT'S YOUR
HEALTH GOAL
FOR THE DAY?:**

_____

WEIGHT:

_____

BMI:

_____

BEDTIME:

_____

Food Log:

Breakfast: _____

_____

_____

Lunch: _____

_____

_____

Dinner: _____

_____

_____

Beverages: _____

_____

Snacks: _____

Notes:

_____

_____

_____

_____

_____

_____

_____

_____

_____

_____

_____

Exercise Log:

Cardio: _____   Time: _____

Distance: _____   Level: _____

Flexibility: _____

Stretches: _____

Classes: _____

Strength: _____   Weight: _____

Repetitions: _____   Sets: _____

✱ Start With a Salad. Or an appetizer like a non-cream-based soup. Those dishes will help you cut calories because you'll eat less of your entrée, says Jonny Bowden, Ph.D., C.N.S., a board-certified nutritionist and author of _The Most Effective Natural Cures on Earth_ (Fair Winds Press). Then you can share your entrée and still feel full.

DATE:

_____

HOURS
OF SLEEP:

_____

HOW
STRESSED
ARE YOU
TODAY? (1-10)

_____

WHAT YOU DID
TO UNWIND:

_____

_____

_____

WHAT'S YOUR
HEALTH GOAL
FOR THE DAY?:

_____

WEIGHT:

_____

BMI:

_____

BEDTIME:

_____

Food Log:

Breakfast: _____
_____
_____

Lunch: _____
_____
_____

Dinner: _____
_____
_____

Beverages: _____
_____

Snacks: _____

Notes:

_____
_____
_____
_____
_____
_____
_____
_____
_____
_____
_____

Exercise Log:

Cardio: _____   Time: _____
Distance: _____   Level: _____

Flexibility: _____
Stretches: _____
Classes: _____

Strength: _____   Weight: _____
Repetitions: _____   Sets: _____

Notes: _____
_____
_____

DATE:

_____

HOURS
OF SLEEP:

_____

HOW
STRESSED
ARE YOU
TODAY? (1-10)

_____

WHAT YOU DID
TO UNWIND:

_____

_____

WHAT'S YOUR
HEALTH GOAL
FOR THE DAY?:

_____

WEIGHT:

_____

BMI:

_____

BEDTIME:

_____

Food Log:

Breakfast: _____
_____
_____

Lunch: _____
_____

Dinner: _____
_____

Beverages: _____

Snacks: _____

Notes:

_____
_____
_____
_____
_____
_____
_____
_____
_____
_____

Exercise Log:

Cardio: _____   Time: _____
Distance: _____   Level: _____

Flexibility: _____
Stretches: _____
Classes: _____

Strength: _____   Weight: _____
Repetitions: _____   Sets: _____

✻Bring Nature Inside. Choose peaceful, earthy hues, like lilac-tinted grays and sea greens, for your home. And opt for touchable, natural fabrics such as silk, fur and cashmere. Bedding made from organic cotton, for example, breathes more and may slow the heart rate and better regulate body temperature, for a good night's sleep.

DATE:

_____

**HOURS
OF SLEEP:**

_____

**HOW
STRESSED
ARE YOU
TODAY? (1-10)**

_____

**WHAT YOU DID
TO UNWIND:**

_____

_____

_____

**WHAT'S YOUR
HEALTH GOAL
FOR THE DAY?:**

_____

WEIGHT:

_____

BMI:

_____

BEDTIME:

_____

Food Log:

Breakfast: _____
_____
_____

Lunch: _____
_____
_____

Dinner: _____
_____
_____

Beverages: _____

Snacks: _____

Notes:

_____
_____
_____
_____
_____
_____
_____
_____

Exercise Log:

Cardio: _____   Time: _____
Distance: _____   Level: _____

Flexibility: _____
Stretches: _____
Classes: _____

Strength: _____   Weight: _____
Repetitions: _____   Sets: _____

Notes: _____
_____
_____

DATE:

_____

**HOURS
OF SLEEP:**

_____

**HOW
STRESSED
ARE YOU
TODAY? (1-10)**

_____

**WHAT YOU DID
TO UNWIND:**

_____

_____

_____

**WHAT'S YOUR
HEALTH GOAL
FOR THE DAY?:**

_____

WEIGHT:

_____

BMI:

_____

BEDTIME:

_____

Food Log:

Breakfast: _____

_____

_____

Lunch: _____

_____

_____

Dinner: _____

_____

_____

Beverages: _____

Snacks: _____

Notes:

_____

_____

_____

_____

_____

_____

_____

_____

_____

_____

Exercise Log:

Cardio: _____   Time: _____

Distance: _____   Level: _____

Flexibility: _____

Stretches: _____

Classes: _____

Strength: _____   Weight: _____

Repetitions: _____   Sets: _____

✱Trim Your Thighs. Try this toning move by celebrity trainer Mark Jenkins: Stand with knees slightly bent and feet apart. Holding a three- or five-pound dumbbell, place left hand over right, squat one third of the way down, squeeze buttocks, and hold for two seconds. Next, squat two thirds of the way down and squeeze. Finally drop into a full squat and squeeze. Return to start. Do three sets of 12.

DATE:

_____

HOURS
OF SLEEP:

_____

HOW
STRESSED
ARE YOU
TODAY? (1-10)

_____

WHAT YOU DID
TO UNWIND:

_____

_____

_____

WHAT'S YOUR
HEALTH GOAL
FOR THE DAY?:

_____

WEIGHT:

_____

BMI:

_____

BEDTIME:

_____

Food Log:

Breakfast: _____

_____

_____

Lunch: _____

_____

_____

Dinner: _____

_____

_____

Beverages: _____

_____

Snacks: _____

Notes:

_____

_____

_____

_____

_____

_____

_____

_____

_____

_____

Exercise Log:

Cardio: _____   Time: _____
Distance: _____   Level: _____

Flexibility: _____
Stretches: _____
Classes: _____

Strength: _____   Weight: _____
Repetitions: _____   Sets: _____

Notes: _____

_____

_____

DATE:

_____

HOURS OF SLEEP:

_____

HOW STRESSED ARE YOU TODAY? (1-10)

_____

WHAT YOU DID TO UNWIND:

_____

_____

_____

WHAT'S YOUR HEALTH GOAL FOR THE DAY?:

_____

WEIGHT:

_____

BMI:

_____

BEDTIME:

_____

Food Log:

Breakfast: _____
_____
_____

Lunch: _____
_____
_____

Dinner: _____
_____
_____

Beverages: _____
_____

Snacks: _____

Notes:

_____
_____
_____
_____
_____
_____
_____
_____
_____

Exercise Log:

Cardio: _____ Time: _____
Distance: _____ Level: _____

Flexibility: _____
Stretches: _____
Classes: _____

Strength: _____ Weight: _____
Repetitions: _____ Sets: _____

✱Talk the Talk. By repeating encouraging affirmations, you can reprogram yourself to see things in a more positive light, says Elizabeth Scott, a family therapist and life coach in Los Angeles. Just make sure your affirmation reflects what you want your reality to be. Instead of saying, _I don't want to feel stress_, say, _I'm feeling peaceful._

COVER

Top Photo: Adam Olszewski Bottom Row (left to right): Digital Vision/Getty Images, Flint/Corbis, Alison Miksch

INTRO

Woman in white dress: Brooke Fasani/Getty Images

PART 1

Body + Soul Opener: John Hicks/Getty Images Healthy at Every Age, 20s: Photodisc/Getty Images Healthy at Every Age, 30s: Bruce Talbot/DK Stock/Getty Images Healthy at Every Age, 40s: Jose Luis Pelaez, Inc./Blend Images/Getty Images Healthy at Every Age, 50s: Peter LaMastro Best Advice, Health Concerns: Tony Hutchings/Photographer's Choice/Getty Images Heart Disease: John Lund/Tiffany Schoepp/Blend Images/Getty Images Ask Yourself: Vincenzo Lombardo/Getty Images If You Do Just One Thing: Ariel Skelley/Getty Images Ask the Docs About Diabetes: Digital Vision/Getty Images

PART 2

Fit + Fabulous Opener: Goodshoot/Corbis 8 Steps to Get You Started: Amana Productions/Getty Images "I Lost With My Family": Credit for both main photos: Sherry Strazis, Before photo: Courtesy of Pamela Williams Surefire Solutions: Lower body picture: Amana Productions, Inc./Getty Images, Bicyclist: Nicole Hill/Getty

Images "I Walked It Off!": Main Photo: Greg Miles, Before Photo: Courtesy of Maleka Beal Total Body Fitness Challenge: Dominic DiSaia/Getty Images 20-Minute Total Body Workout: Credit for all images: Adam Olszewski Pilates: Credit for all images: Adam Olszewski Armed + Fabulous: Credit for all images: Adam Olszewski Bring Up the Rear: Credit for all images: Adriano Fagundes Gentle Moves: Credit for all images: Adam Olszewski

PART 3

Mind + Spirit Opener: Bambu Productions/Getty Images Just Say Aahhh!: Thomas M. Barwick/Getty Images Aromatherapy: Seth Joel/Getty Images Meditation: Jack Hollingsworth/Getty Images Reflexology: Chromacome/Getty Images Acupuncture: Jon Feingersh/Getty Images Massage: Jon Feingersh/Getty Image Deep Stretch Yoga: Woman on floor: John Giustina/Getty Images, Woman outside: Flint/Corbis African Dance: Steve Vaccariello/Getty Images Your Pursuit of Happiness: Sandra Seckinger/Zefa/Corbis Is It More Than Just the Blues?: Robin Lynne Gibson How to Pray: Gary Parker/Getty Images

PART 4

Sexual Health Opener: Dagmara The Vagina Dialogues: Laureen March/Corbis Safe Safe Sex 101: Digital Vision/Getty Images Fibroids: Davies

and Starr/Getty Images Your Most Intimate Questions, Answered: Art Vandalay/Getty Images Sexy at Every Age, 20s: Ryan Mcvay/Getty Images Sexy at Every Age, 30s: Russell Sadur/Getty Images Sexy at Every Age, 40s: Digital Vision/Getty Images Sexy at Every Age, 50s: Robert Kent Canada, Inc./Getty Images

PART 5

Healthy Food Fast Opener: Noel Hendrickson/Getty Images Servin' It Up!: Photography, Jim Franco. Food Stylist, Susan Ottaviano. Prop Stylist, Paul Lowe. Foods That Energize: Stockbyte/Getty Images Chicken With Lemon–Pepper Sauce: Jennifer Levy Jerk Turkey burger: James Baigrie Pepper-Crusted Grouper: James Baigrie Seared Scallops: Alison Miksch Tex-Mex Taco Salad: Jennifer Levy Spicy Kebobs: Alison Miksch Polenta + Summer Vegetables: Alison Miksch Brown Rice + Sautéed Vegetables: Beatriz da Costa Oatmeal With Dried Cherries: Beatriz da Costa Summer Fruit Shortcake: Alison Miksch Spicy Shrimp With Grits: Frances Janisch Baked Macaroni + Cheese: Ann Stratton Nourish Your Body at Every Age: John Giustina/Getty Images

PART 6

Healthy Living Journal, Start Your Journey: Plush Studios/Getty Images